Alkaline Smoothies

50 Recipes for Your Everyday Alkaline Smoothie

Naomi Whiteley

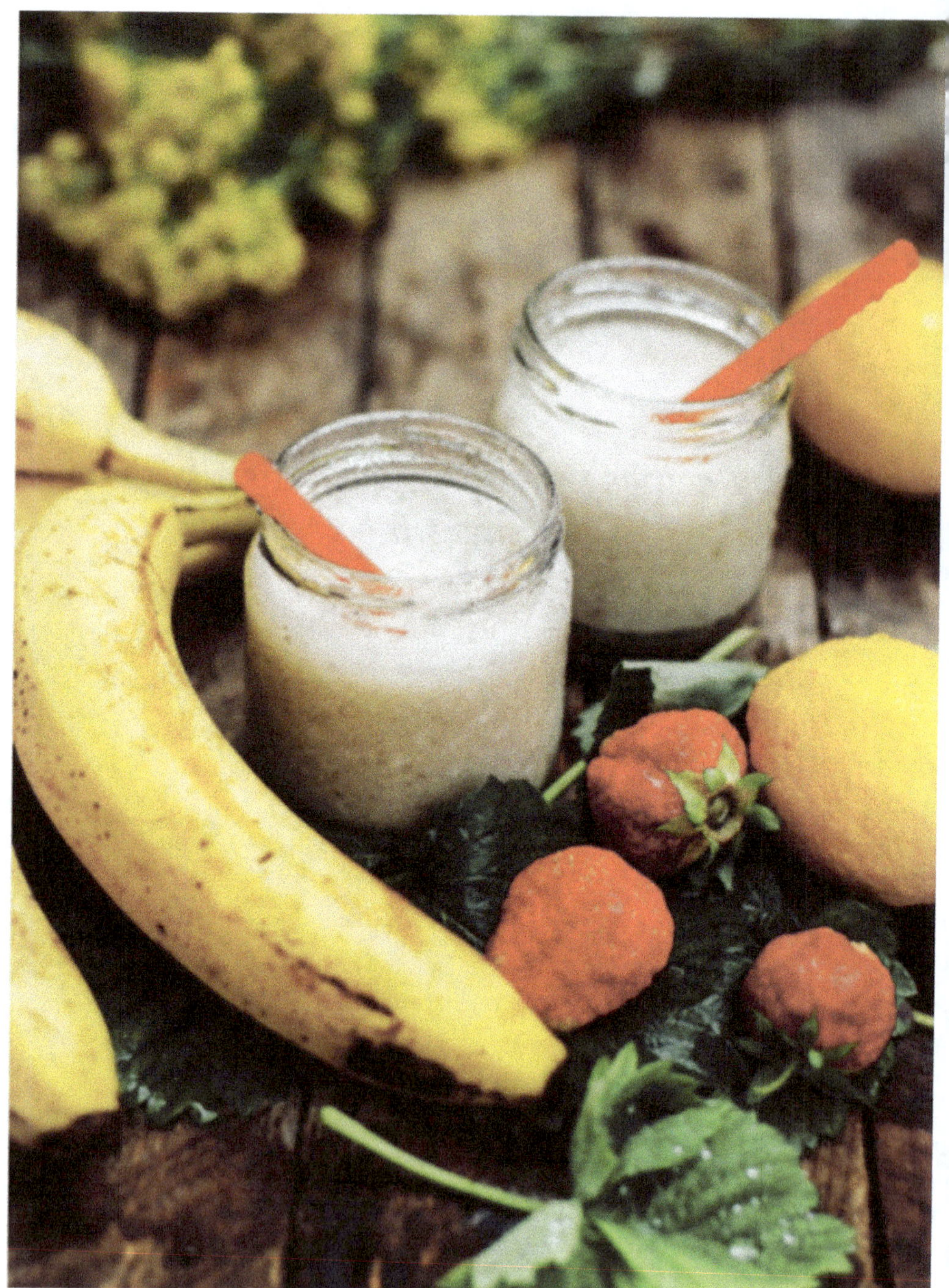

professional before attempting any techniques outlined in this book.

By reading this document, the reader agrees that under no circumstances is the author responsible for any losses, direct or indirect, which are incurred as a result of the use of information contained within this document, including, but not limited to, — errors, omissions, or inaccuracies.

Table of Contents

Vegetable Freshness

Ingredients:

Tomato (Cherry and plum only), 1/2 cup

1 Cucumber

1 Bell Peppers

Pure Sea Salt to taste

Instructions:

1.   Cut all vegetables for the blender.

2.   Blend all ingredients in a high-speed blender until smooth.

3.   Enjoy!

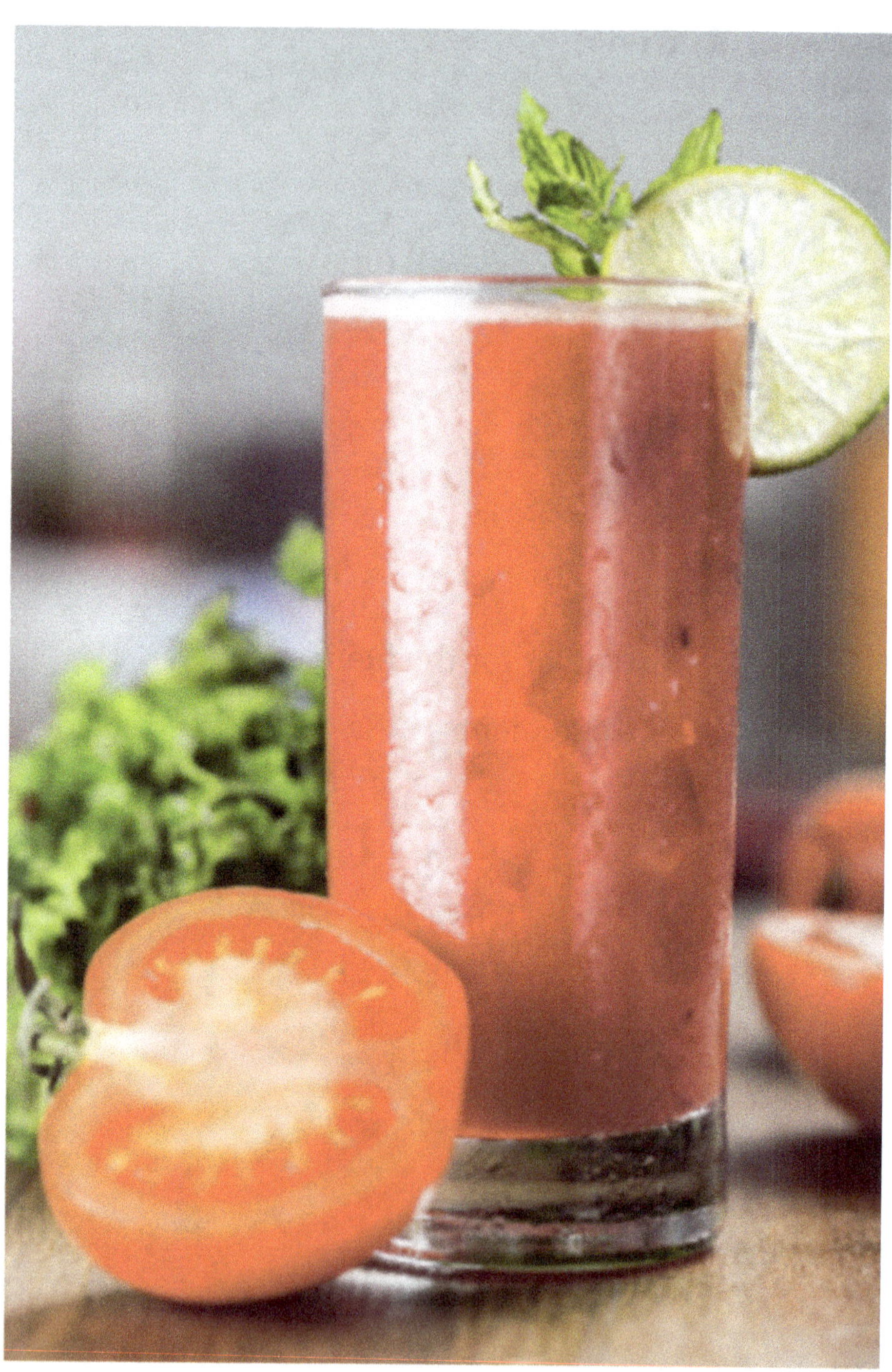

Antioxidant Smoothie

Ingredients:

Zucchini, 1 (medium size)

Date Sugar, 2 teaspoons

Instructions:

1.   Cut zucchini for the blender.

2.   Blend all ingredients in a high-speed blender until smooth.

3.   Enjoy!

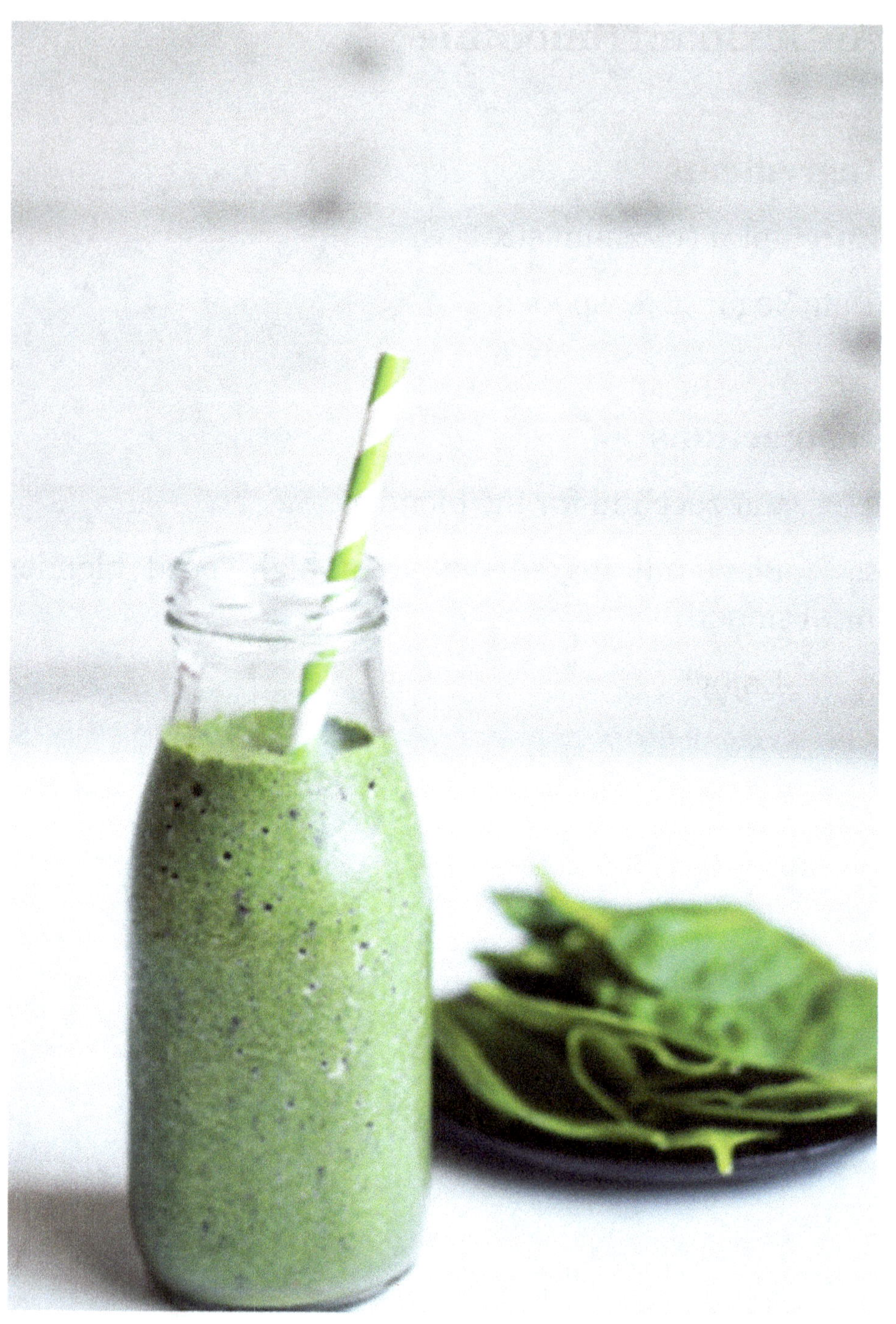

Multi Berries Smoothie

Ingredients:

Soft Jelly Coconut Milk (or homemade walnut milk)

½ cup

Date Sugar

2 teaspoons

1 Banana (The smallest one or the Burro/ midsize/ original banana)

Blueberries/Blackberries/Raspberries (or mix)

½ cup

Instructions:

1.	Blend all ingredients in a high-speed blender until smooth.

2.	Enjoy!

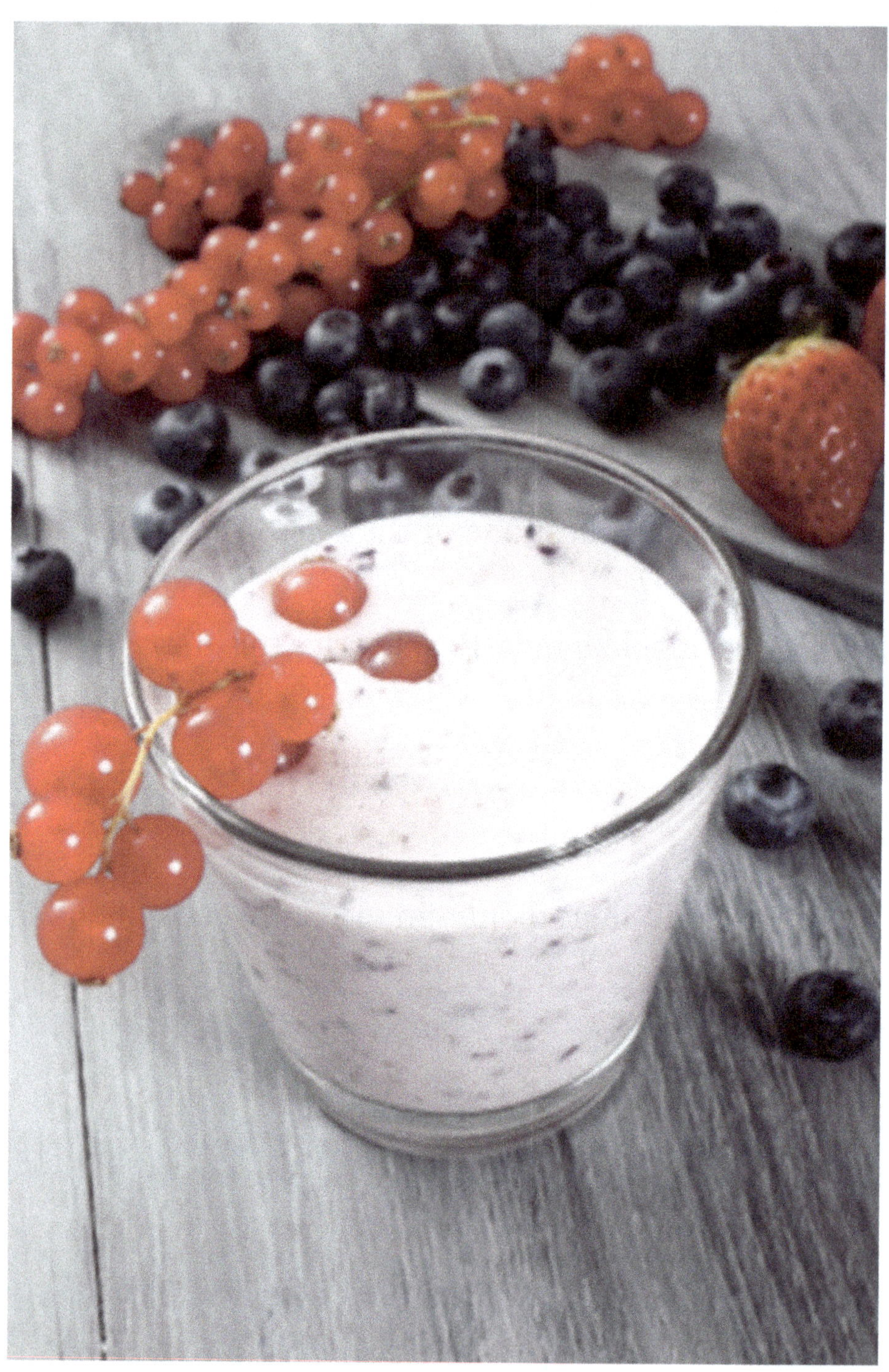

Spicy Cucumber Smoothie

Ingredients:

Cucumber Ginger, grated

4 (medium size)

¼ teaspoons

Instructions:

1.   Cut cucumbers for the blender.

2.   Blend all ingredients in a high-speed blender until smooth.

3.   Enjoy!

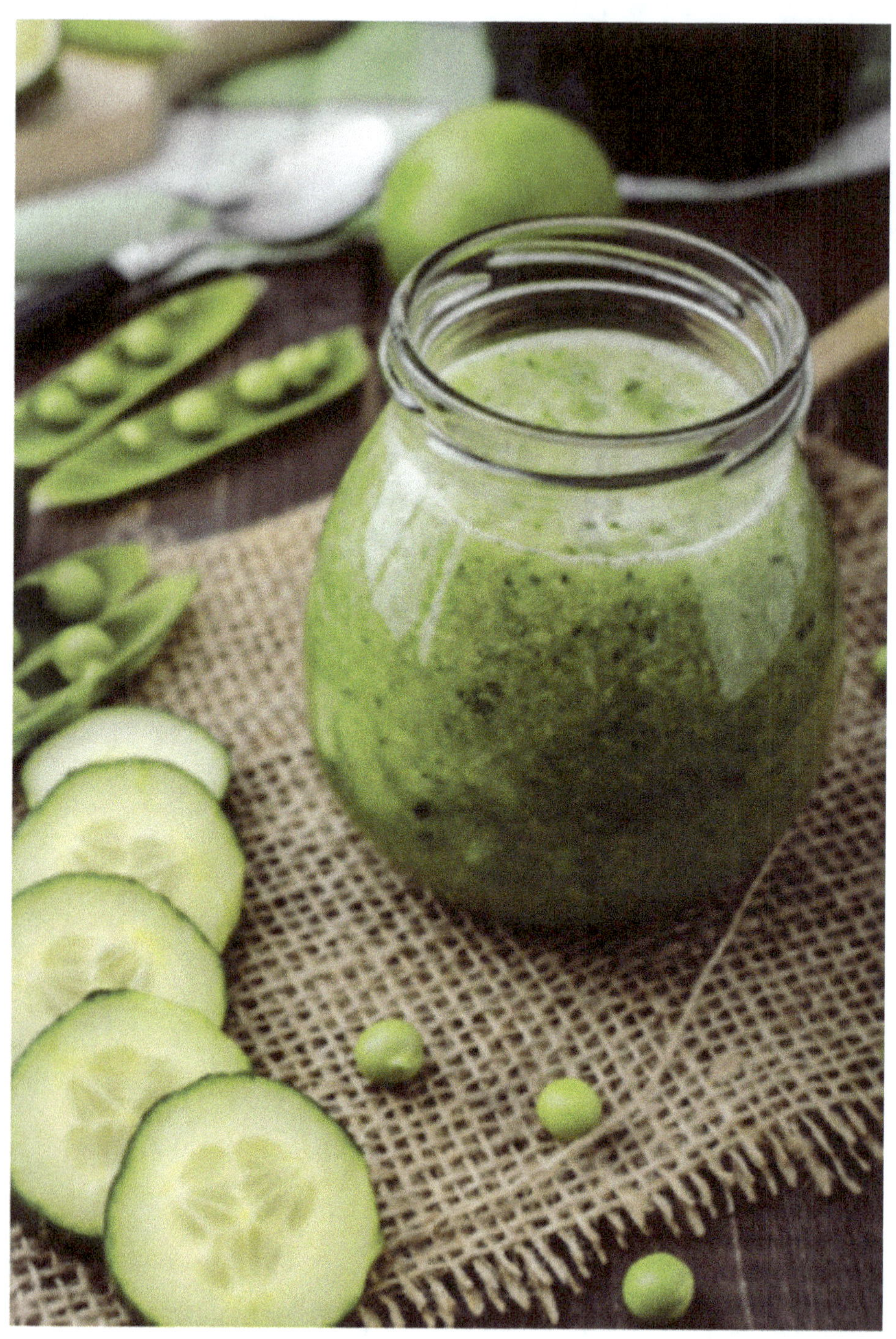

Vegetable Packed Smoothie

Ingredients:

1/2 cup Tomato (Cherry and plum only)

2 Cucumbers

1 Onion

Pure Sea Salt to taste

Instructions:

1.   Cut all vegetables for the blender.

2.   Blend all ingredients in a high-speed blender until smooth.

3.   Enjoy!

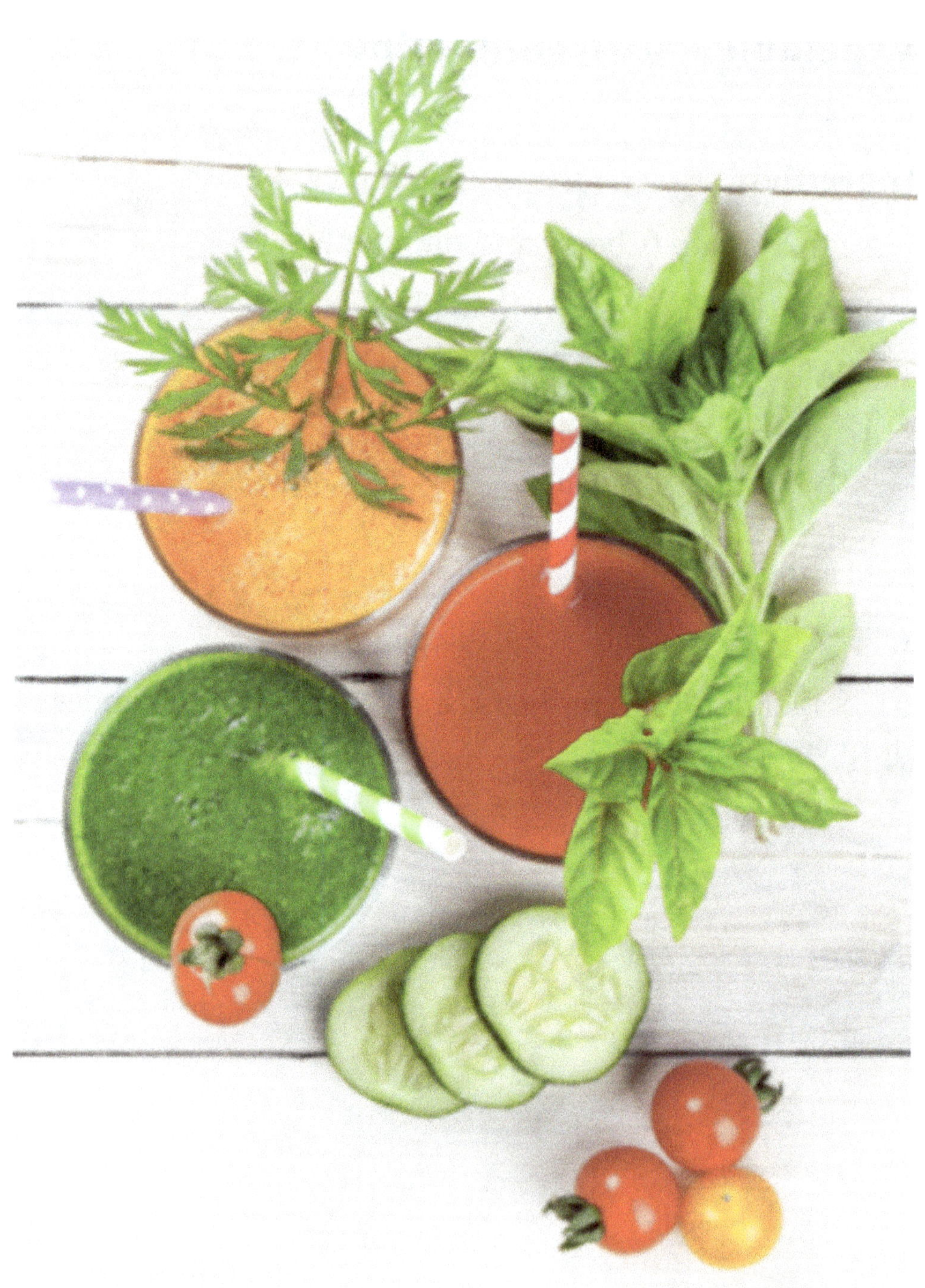

Date Smoothie

Ingredients:

½ cup Soft Jelly Coconut Milk (or homemade walnut milk)

Dates, pitted ¼ cup

1 Bananas (The smallest one or the Burro/midsize/original banana)

Instructions:

1. Cut banana for the blender.

2. Blend all ingredients in a high-speed blender until smooth.

3. Enjoy!

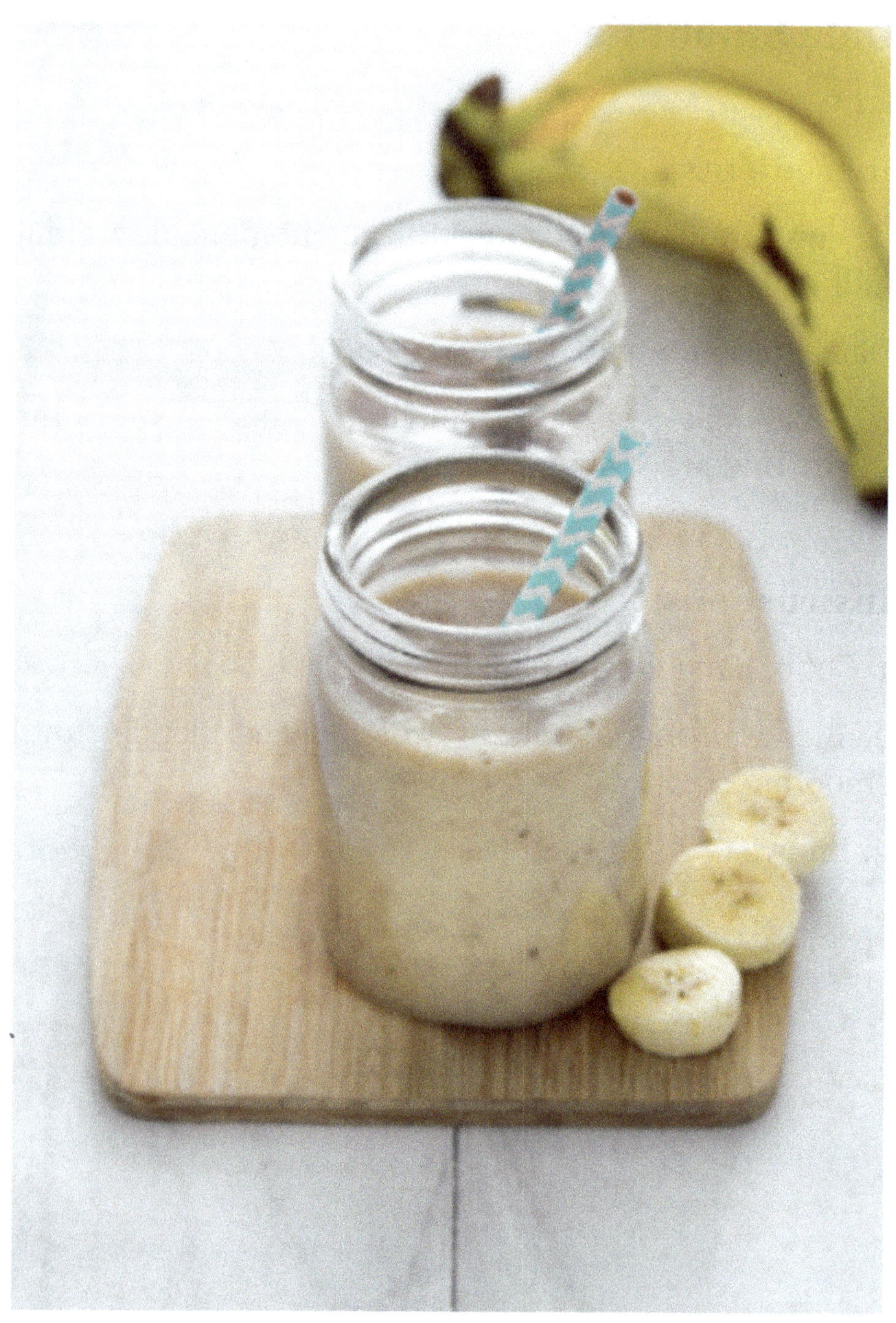

Banana Smoothie

Ingredients:

½ cup Soft Jelly Coconut Milk (or homemade walnut milk)

2 teaspoons Date Sugar

About ½ cup Bananas (The smallest one or the Burro/midsize/original banana)

Instructions:

1. Cut bananas for the blender.

2. Blend all ingredients in a high-speed blender until smooth.

3. Enjoy!

Anti-Bacteria Smoothie

Ingredients:

Soft Jelly Coconut Milk (or homemade walnut milk), ½ cup

Date Sugar, 2 teaspoons

Ginger, grated, ¼ teaspoons

Soursops, pitted, peeled, ½ cup

Instructions:

1.   Cut soursops for the blender.

2.   Blend all ingredients in a high-speed blender until smooth.

3.   Pour the mixture into a nut milk bag.

4.   Enjoy!

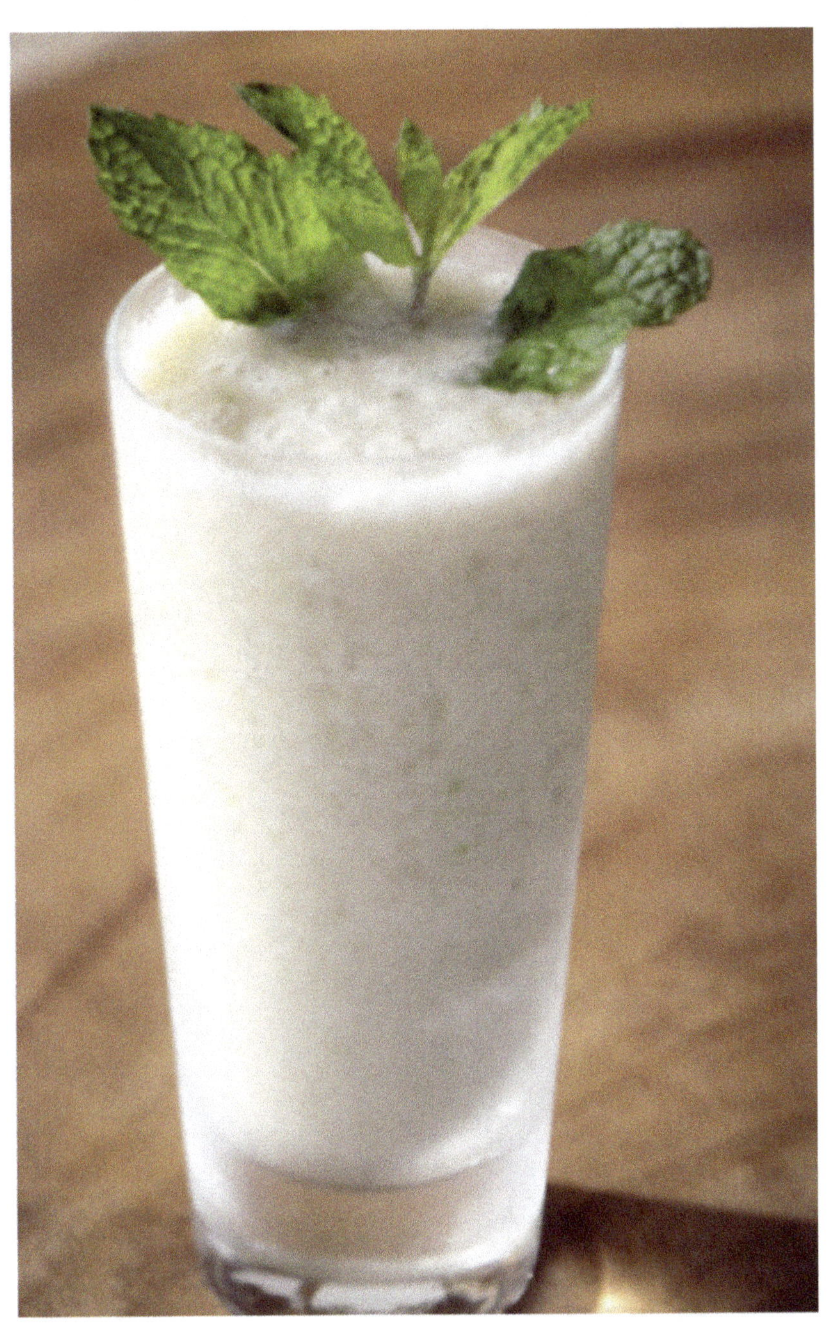

Summer Snack Smoothie

Ingredients:

Soft Jelly Coconut Milk (or homemade walnut milk), ¼ cup

Date Sugar, 2 teaspoons

Cherry, 1/3 cup

Strawberries, 1/3 cup

Instructions:

1.   Blend all ingredients in a high-speed blender until smooth.

2.   Enjoy!

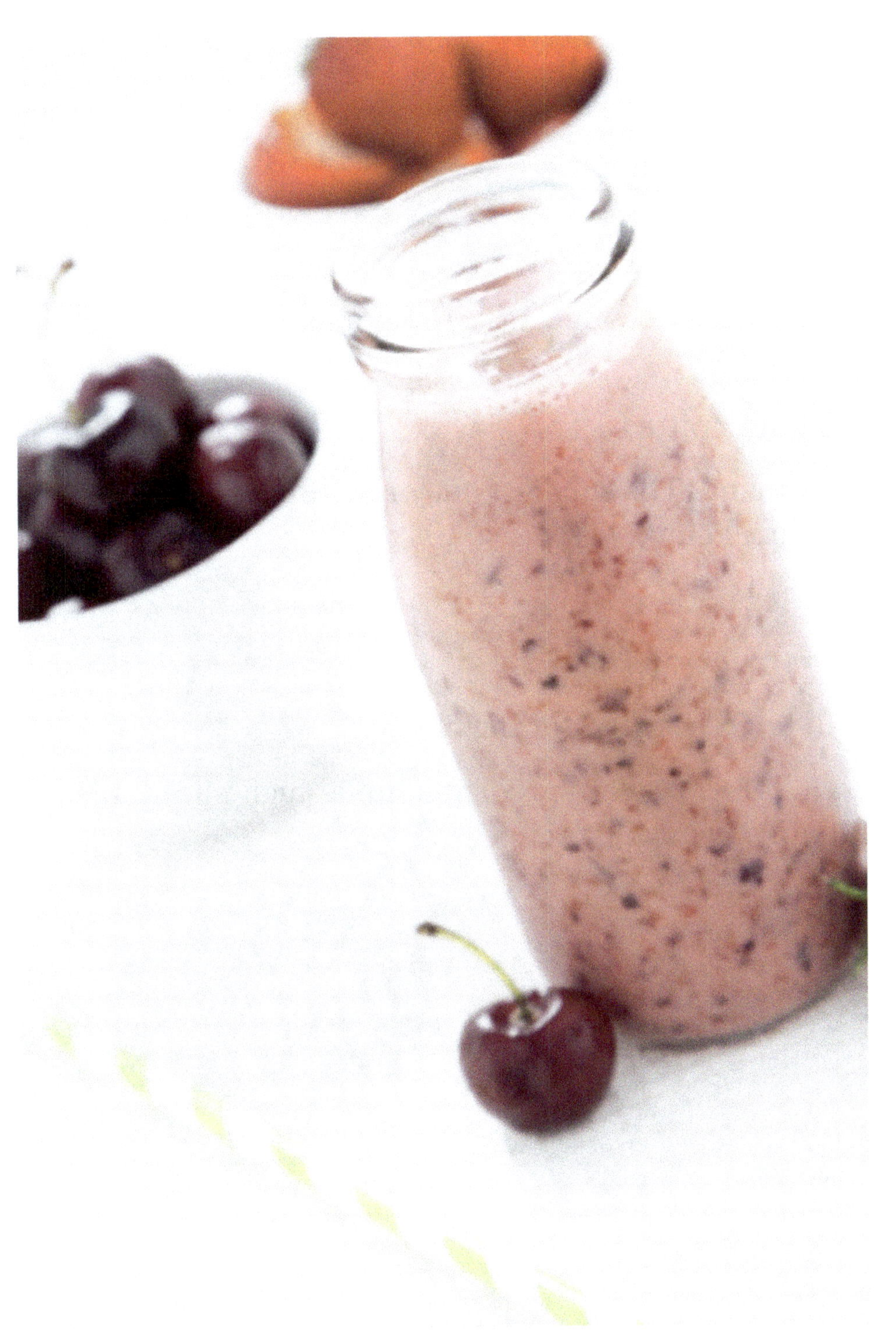

Spelt Smoothie

Ingredients:

Spelt, cooked, ¼ cup

Soft Jelly Coconut Milk (or homemade walnut milk), ½ cup

5 Dates, pitted

1 Banana (The smallest one or the Burro/ midsize/ original banana)

Instructions:

1.   Cut banana for the blender.

2.   Blend all ingredients in a high-speed blender until smooth.

3.   Enjoy!

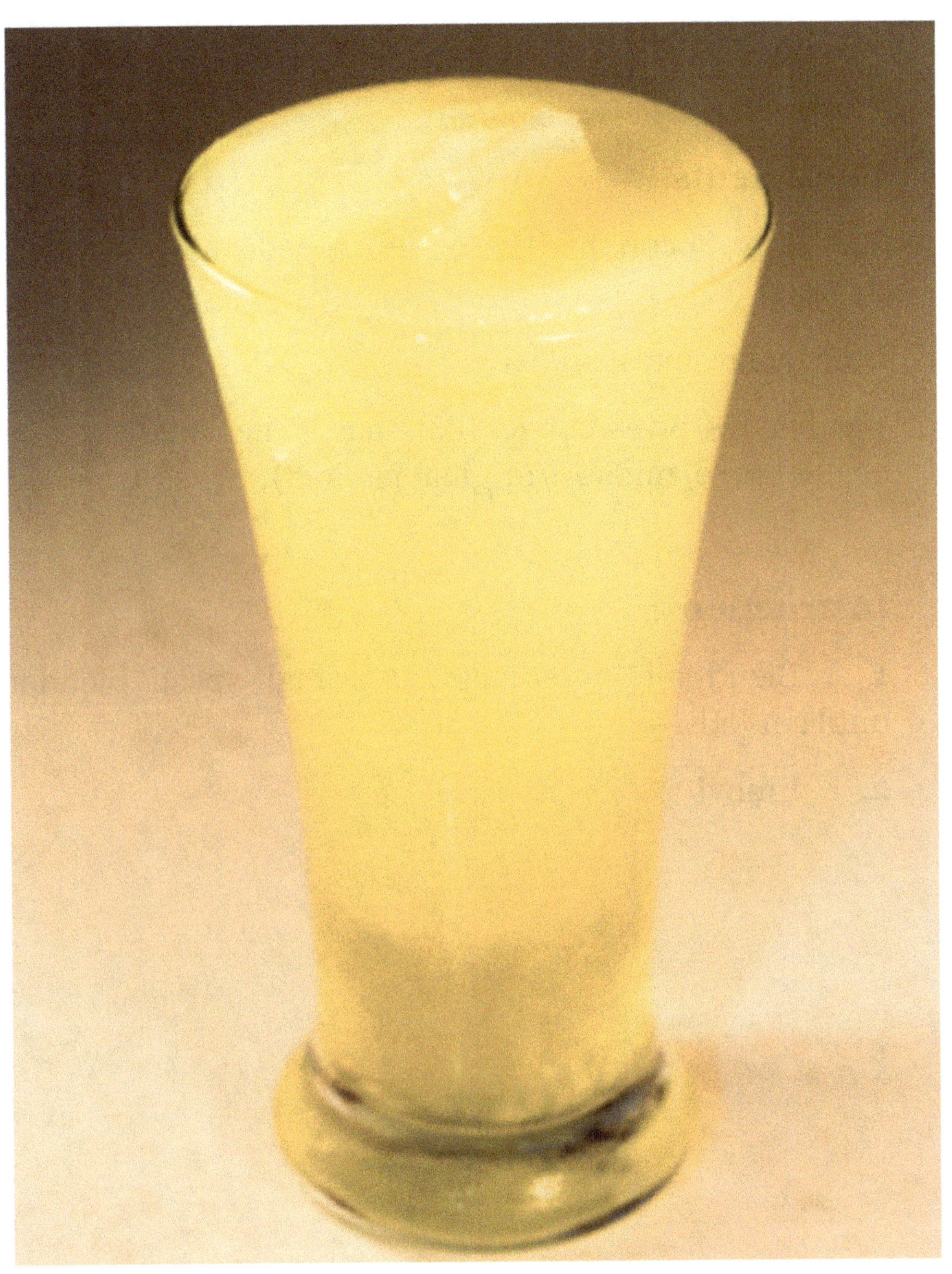

Milky Smoothie

Ingredients:

Soft Jelly Coconut Milk (or homemade walnut milk), 2/3 cup

Date Sugar, 2 teaspoons

Blueberries/Strawberries/Bananas (The smallest one or the Burro/midsize/original banana), 1/3 cup

Instructions:

1.   Blend all ingredients in a high-speed blender until smooth.

2.   Enjoy!

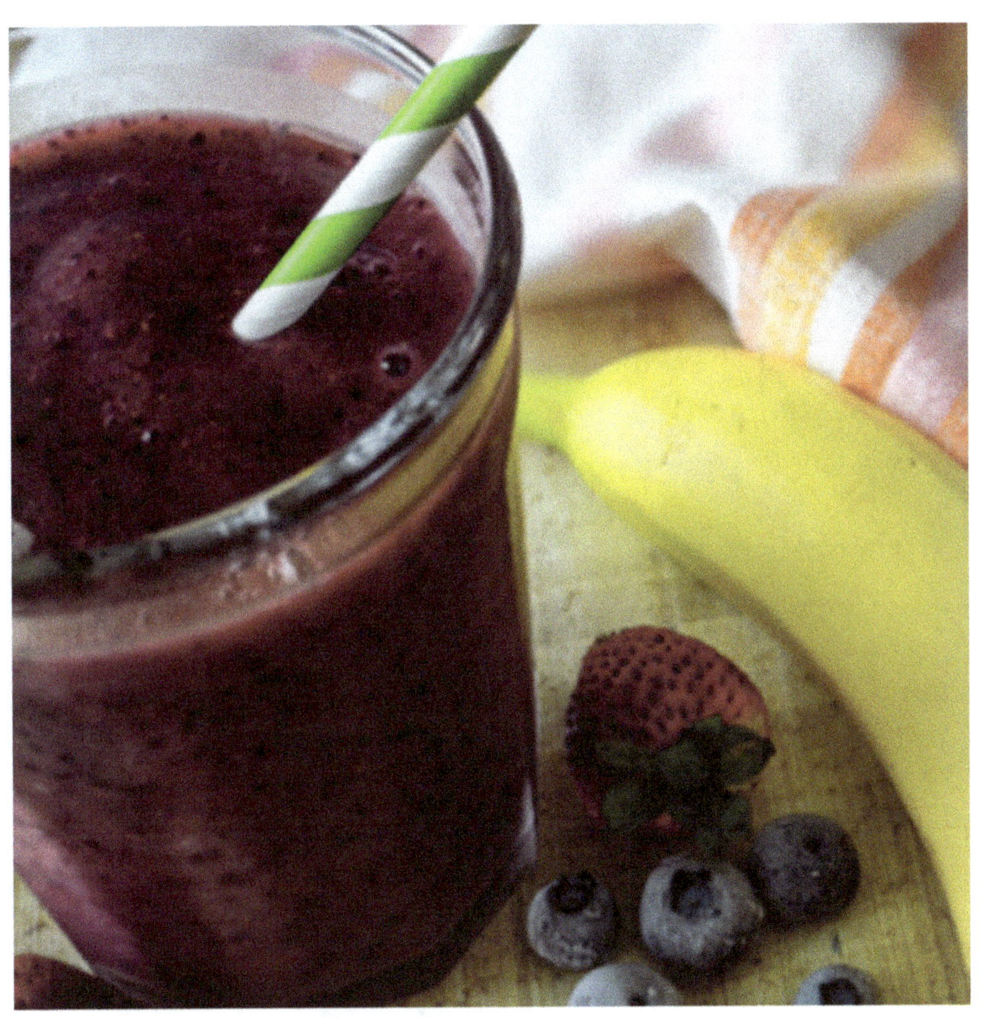

Banana and Strawberry Smoothie

Ingredients:

Soft Jelly Coconut Milk (or homemade walnut milk), ½ cup

Date Sugar, 2 teaspoons

Strawberries, ¼ cup

1 Banana (The smallest one or the Burro/ midsize/ original banana)

Instructions:

1.   Cut bananas for the blender.

2.   Blend all ingredients in a high-speed blender until smooth.

3.   Enjoy!

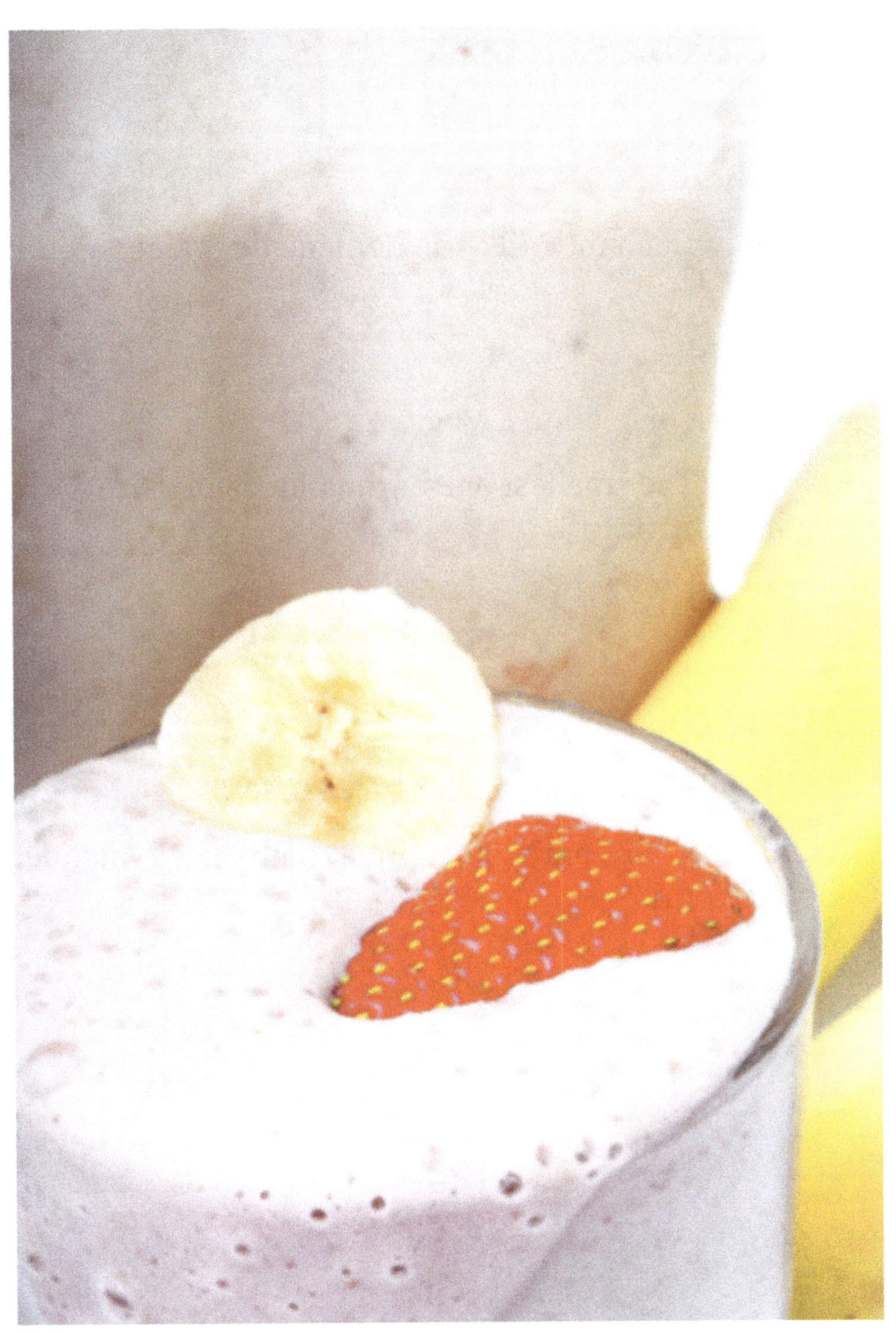

Fig and Nut Smoothie

Ingredients:

Soft Jelly Coconut Milk (or homemade walnut milk), ¼ cup

2, Figs, peeled

Brazil Nuts or Walnuts, ¼ cup

1 Banana (The smallest one or the Burro/ midsize/ original banana)

Instructions:

1.   Cut figs and banana for the blender.

2.   Blend all ingredients in a high-speed blender until smooth.

3.   Enjoy!

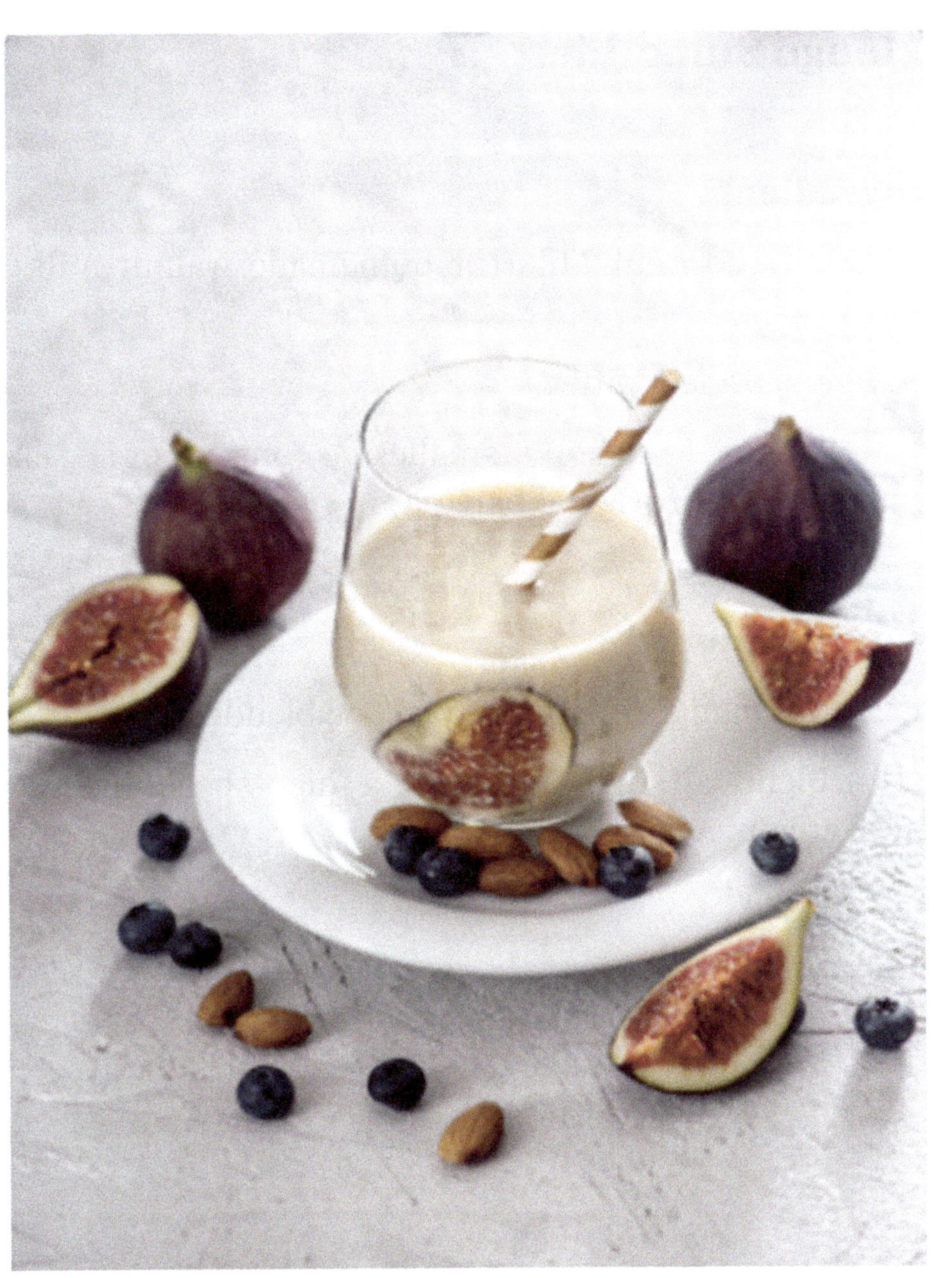

Mango Smoothie

Ingredients:

Soft Jelly Coconut Milk (or homemade walnut milk), ½ cup

1 Mango, peeled, pitted

1 Banana (The smallest one or the Burro/midsize/original banana)

Instructions:

1. Cut mango and banana for the blender.

2. Blend all ingredients in a high-speed blender until creamy.

3. Enjoy!

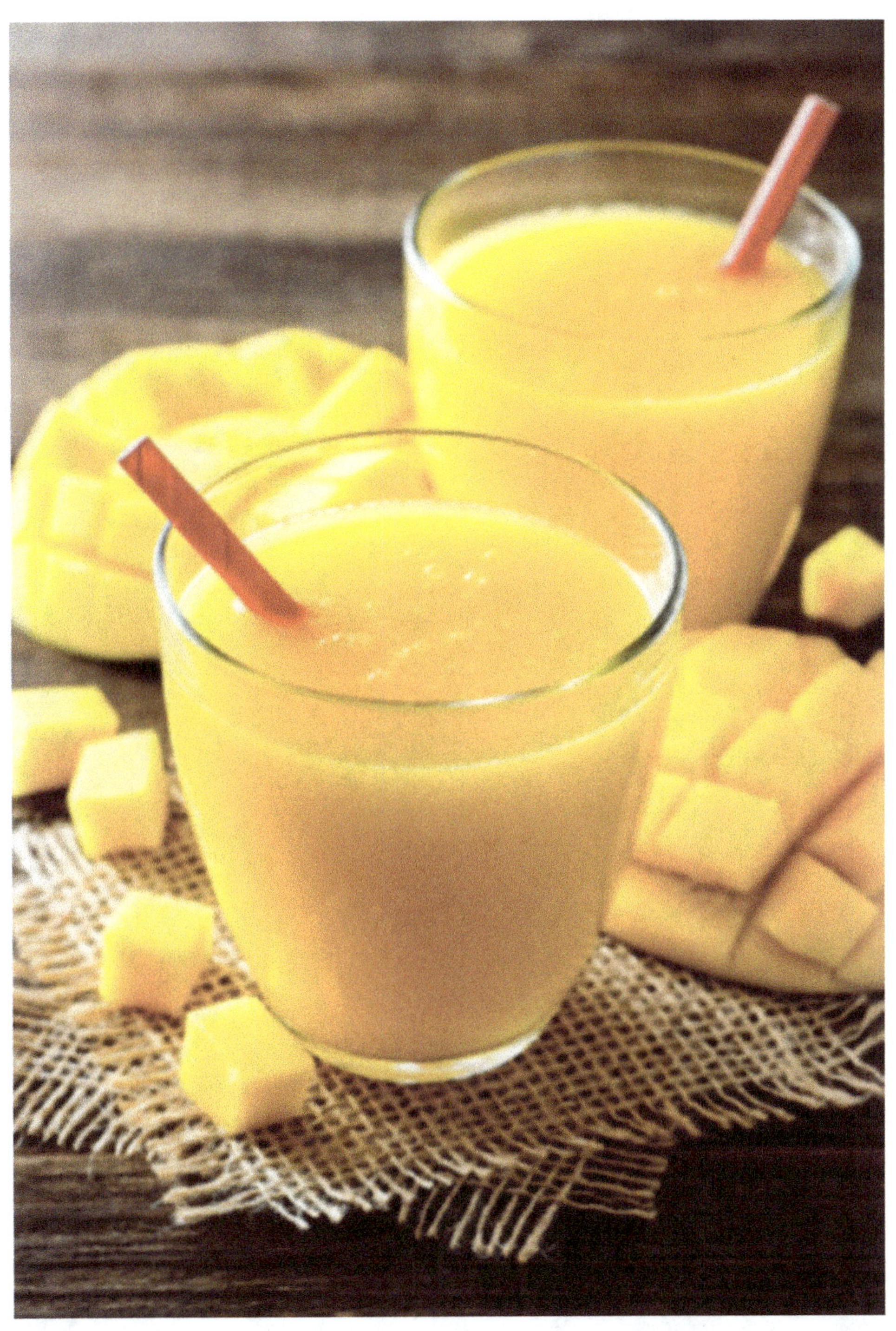

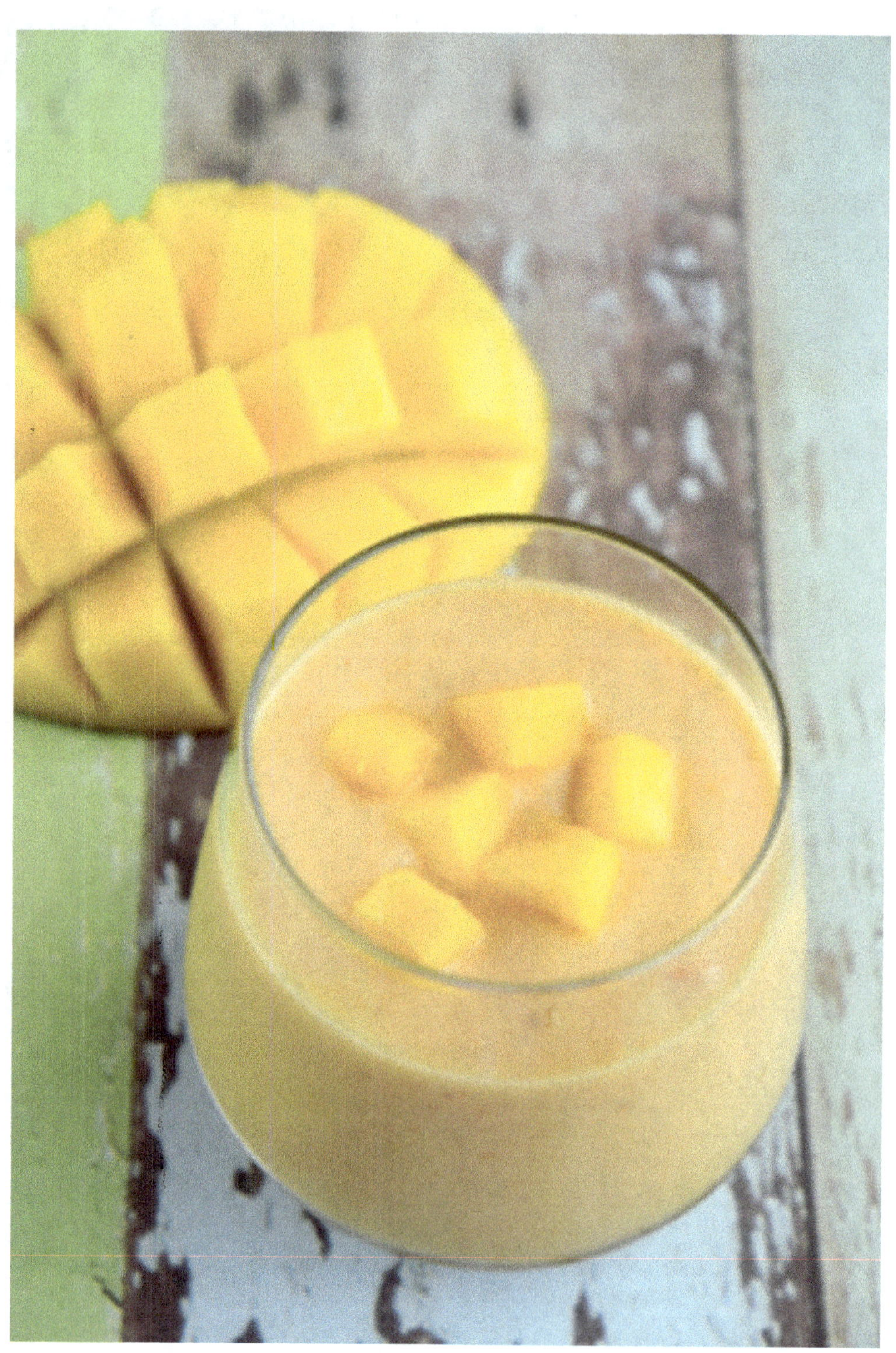

Soft Fig Smoothie

Ingredients:

½ cup, Soft Jelly Coconut Milk (or homemade walnut milk)

4 Figs, peeled

Instructions:

1.   Cut figs for the blender.

2.   Blend all ingredients in a high-speed blender until creamy.

3.   Enjoy!

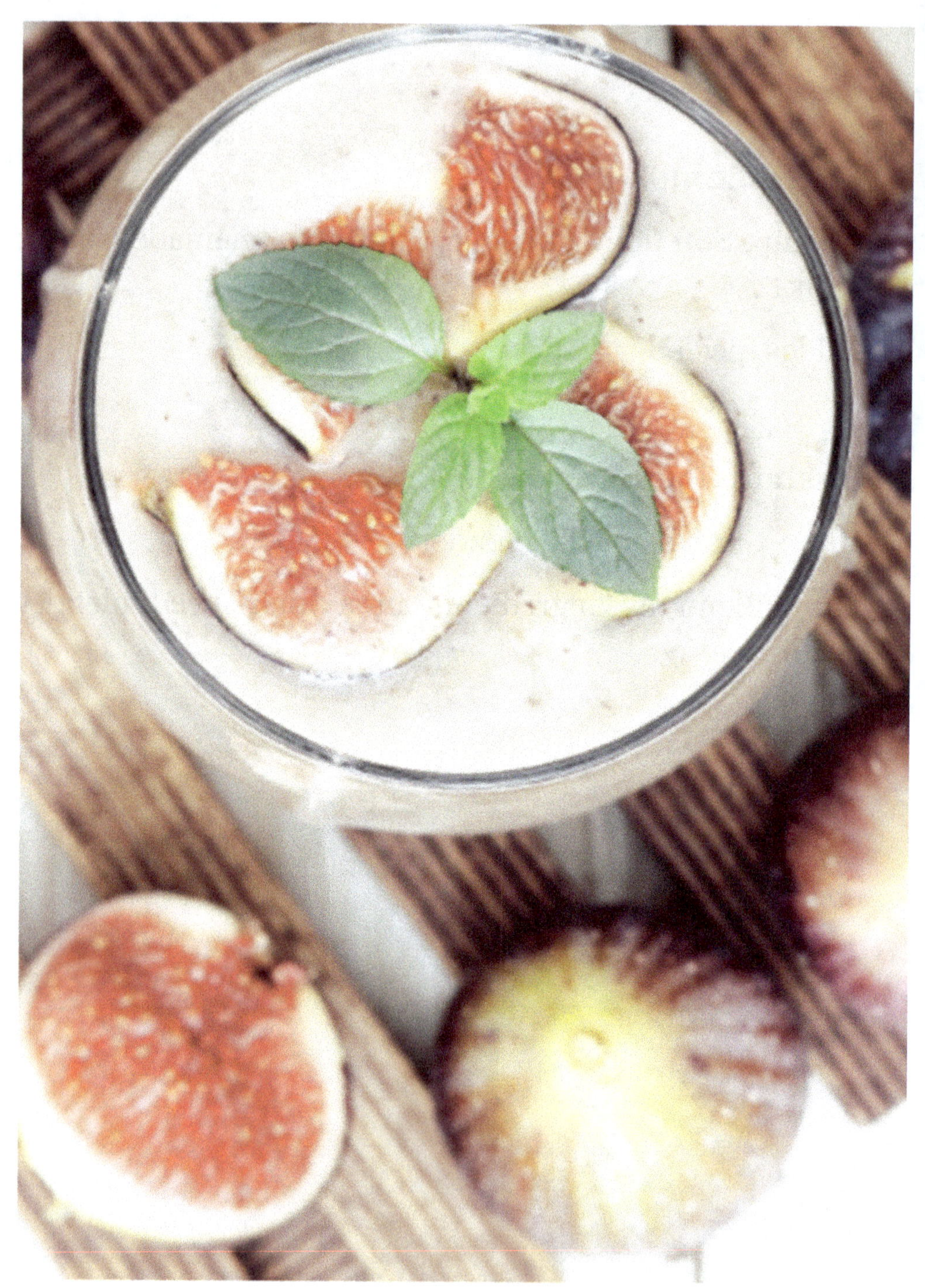

Amaranth Smoothie

Ingredients:

Soft Jelly Coconut Milk (or homemade walnut milk), ½ cup

Amaranth greens, ½ cup

Date Sugar, 2 teaspoons

Sage or Thyme, ¼ teaspoon

Instructions:

1.   Blend all ingredients in a high-speed blender until smooth.

2.   Enjoy!

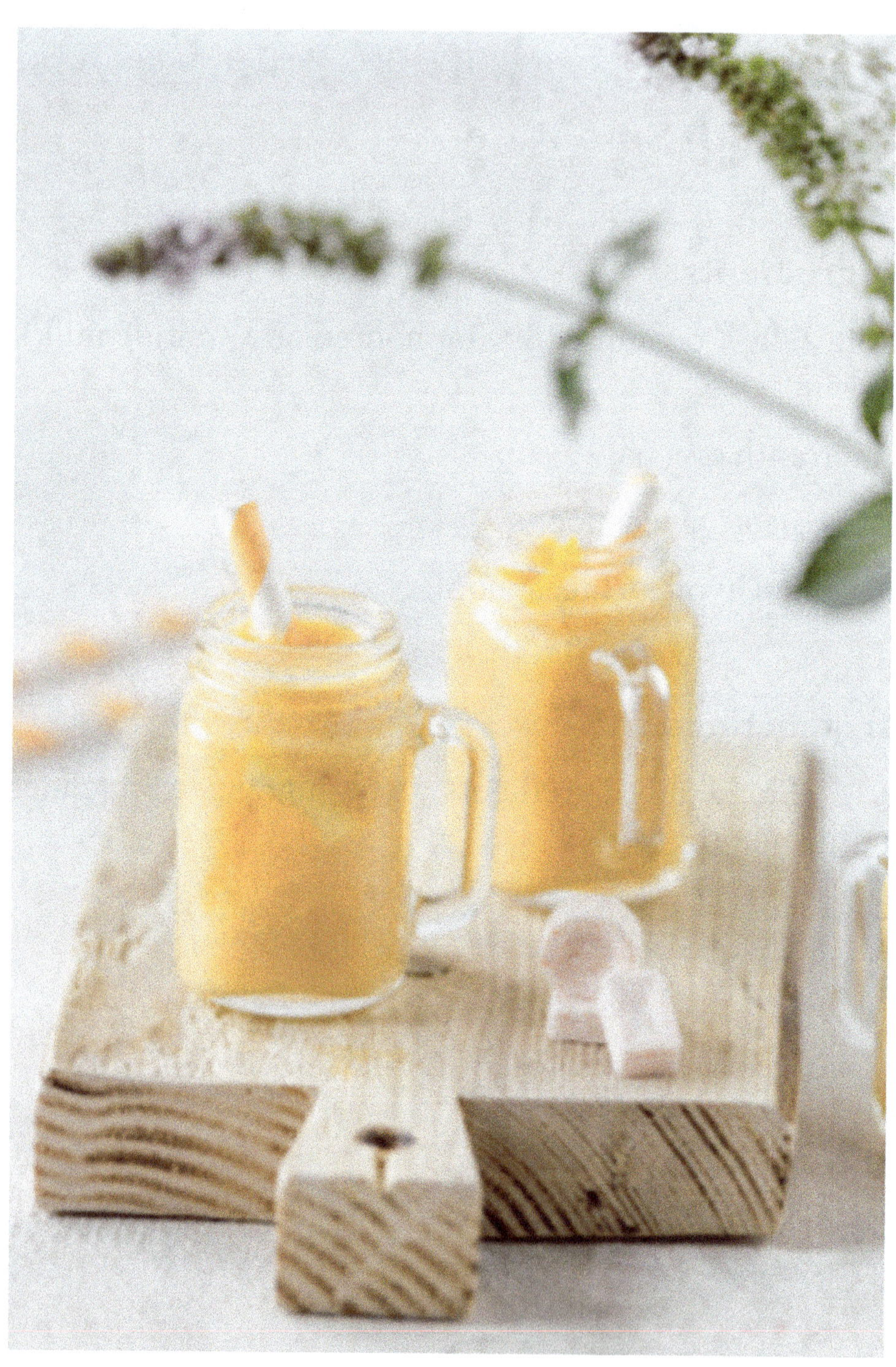

Grape Smoothie

Ingredients:

Grapes (Seeded), 1 cup

Ginger, grated 1 teaspoon

Instructions:

1.   Blend all ingredients in a high-speed blender until smooth.

2.   Enjoy!

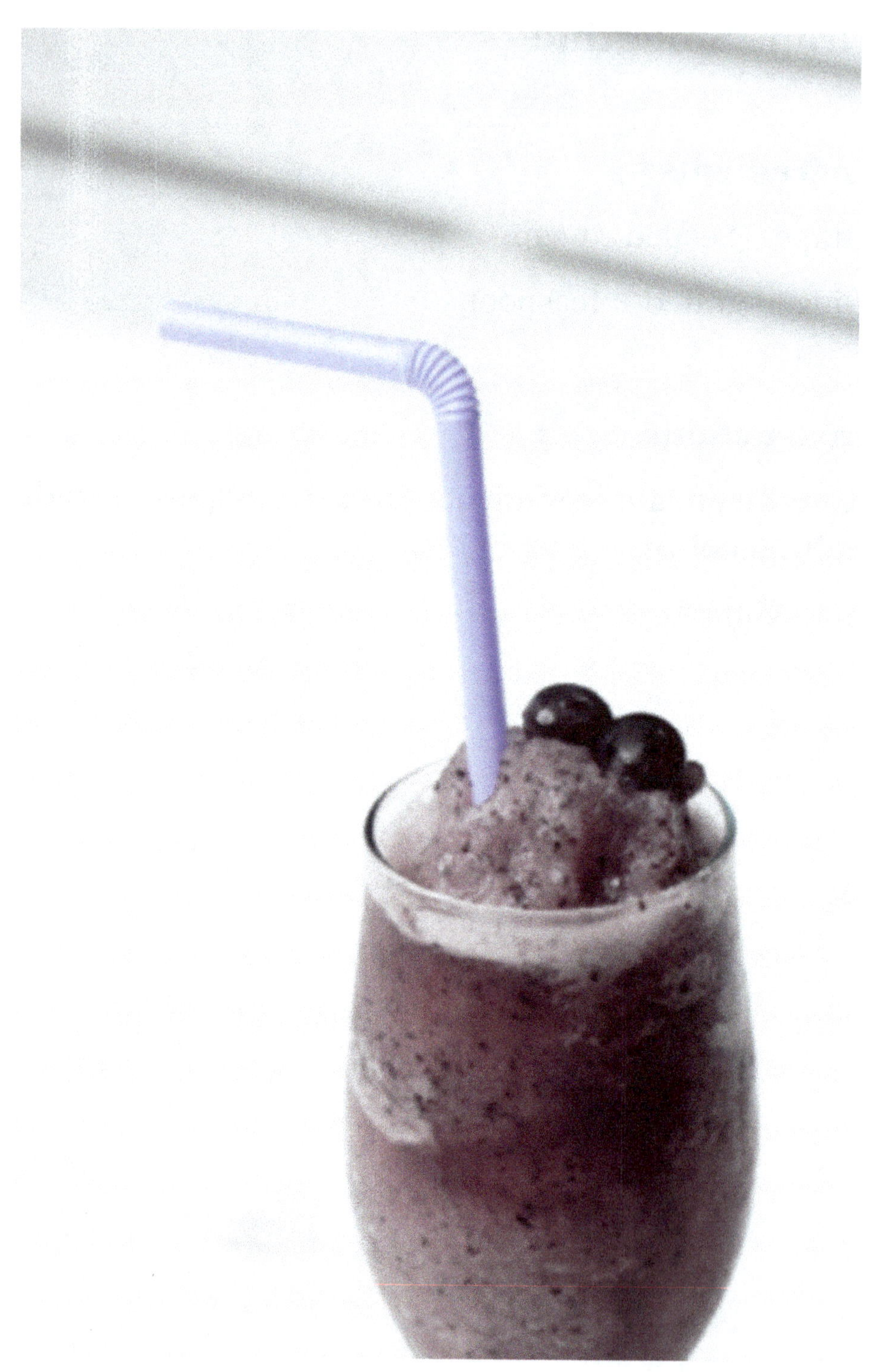

Kale Smoothie

Ingredients:

Chamomile tea, ½ cup

Kale leaves, ½ cup

Date Sugar, 2 teaspoons

1 Banana (The smallest one or the Burro/ midsize/ original banana)

Instructions:

1. Boil ½ cup of water. Add ½ teaspoon of chamomile and let it steep for 10-15 minutes.

2. Strain and let it cool.

3. Cut banana and kale leaves for the blender.

4. Blend all ingredients in a high-speed blender until smooth.

5. Add tea and pulse one more time until mix well.

6. Enjoy!

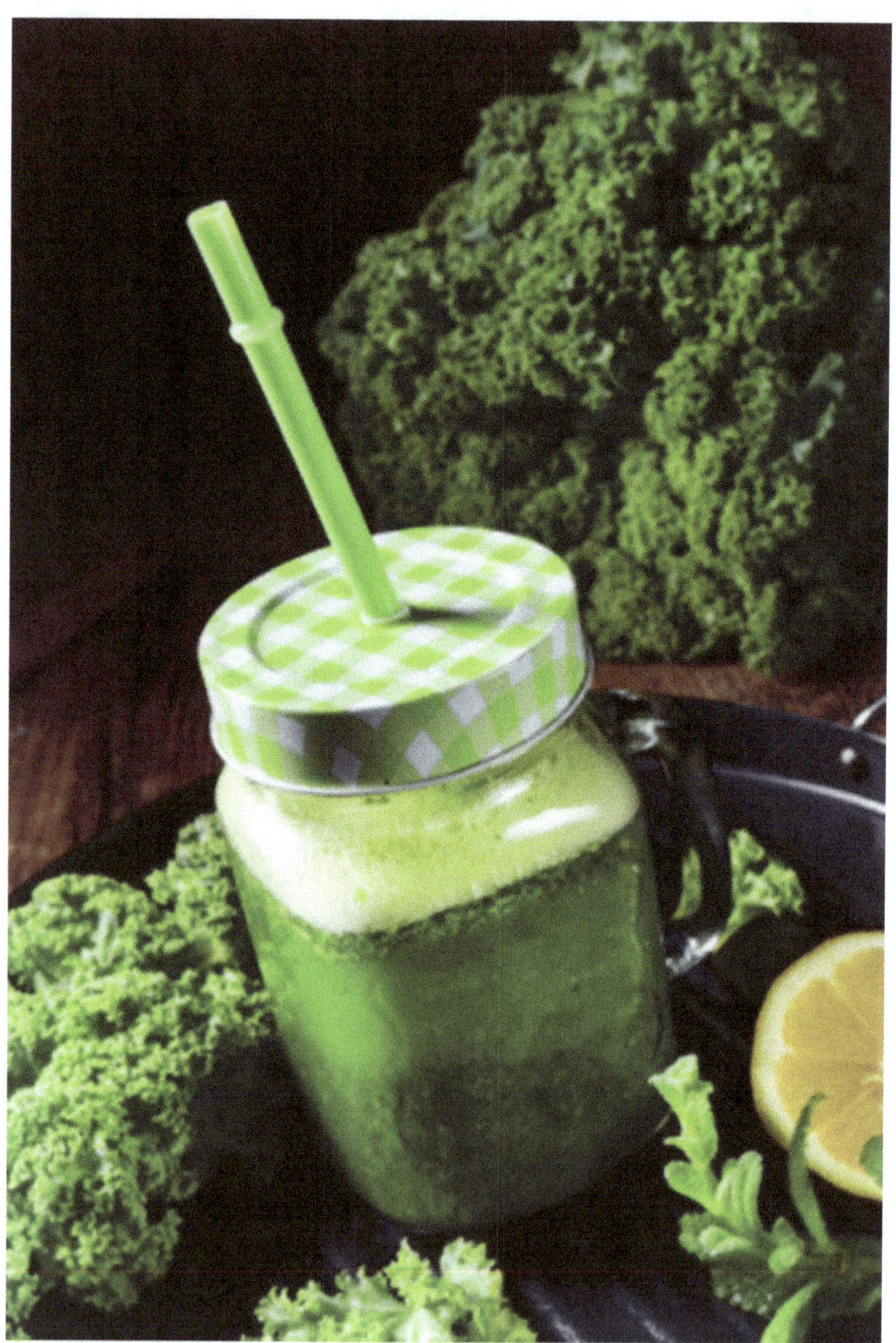

Apple Smoothie

Ingredients:

3 Apples, pitted

Pure Agave Syrup (From cactus) or Date Sugar, 2 teaspoons

(Optional) Brazil Nuts or Walnuts, ¼ cup

Instructions:

1.   Cut apples for the blender.

2.   Blend all ingredients in a high-speed blender until smooth.

3.   Enjoy!

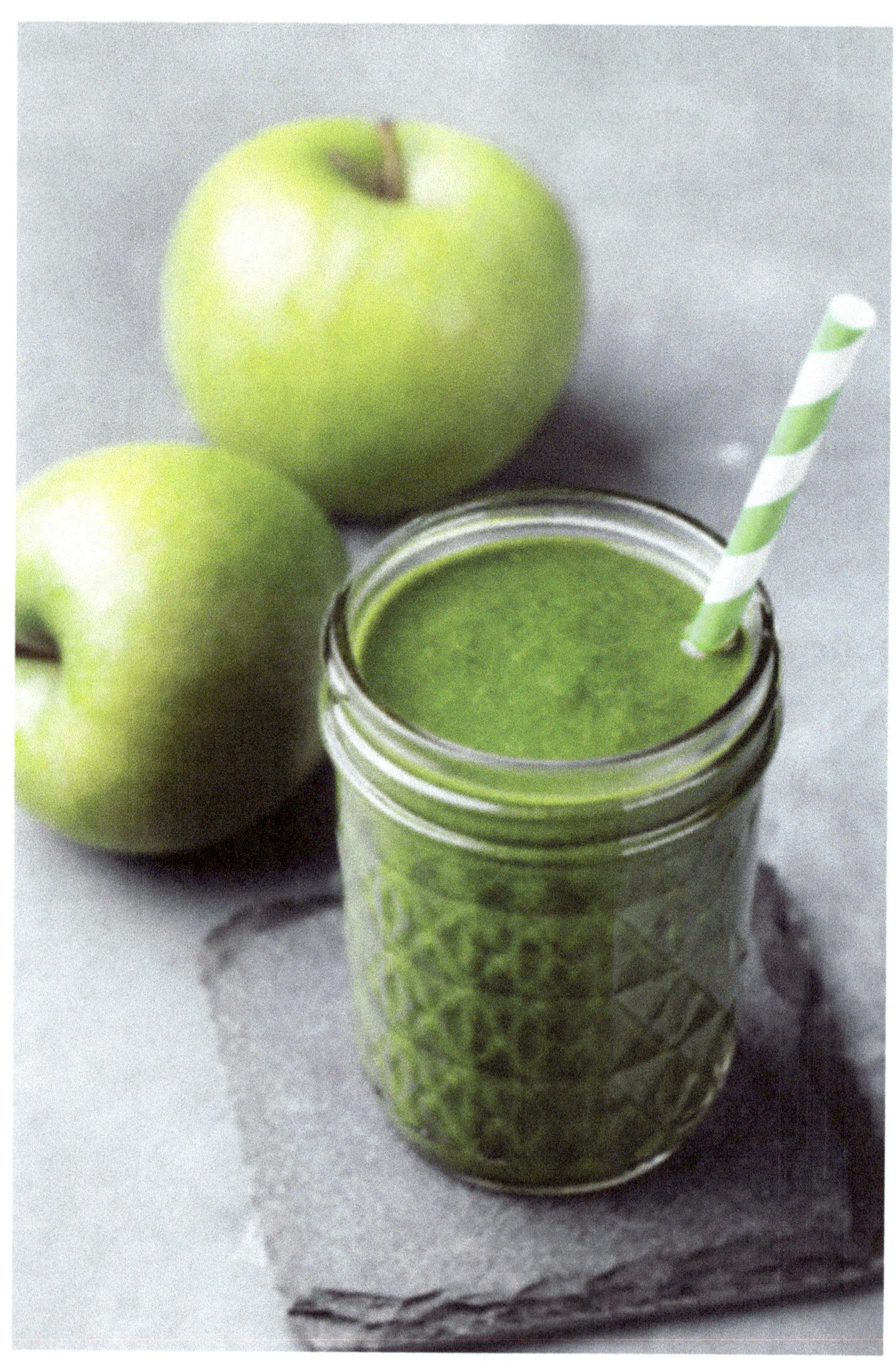

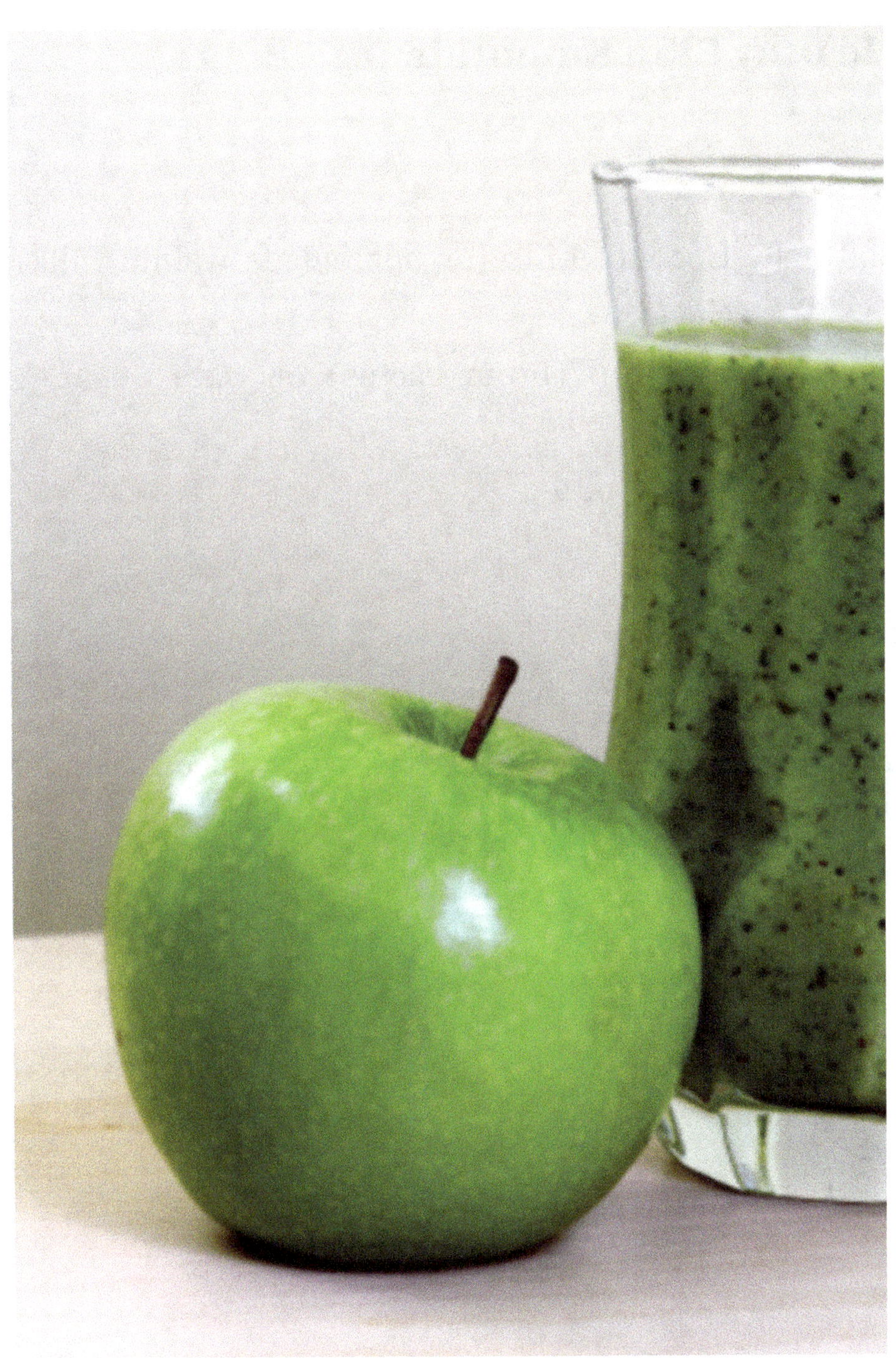

Healthy Skin Smoothie

Ingredients:

Soft Jelly Coconut Milk (or homemade walnut milk), ½ cup

Pure Agave Syrup (From cactus) or Date Sugar, 2 teaspoons

1 Orange, peeled, pitted

Instructions:

1.   Cut orange for the blender.

2.   Blend all ingredients in a high-speed blender until creamy.

3.   Enjoy!

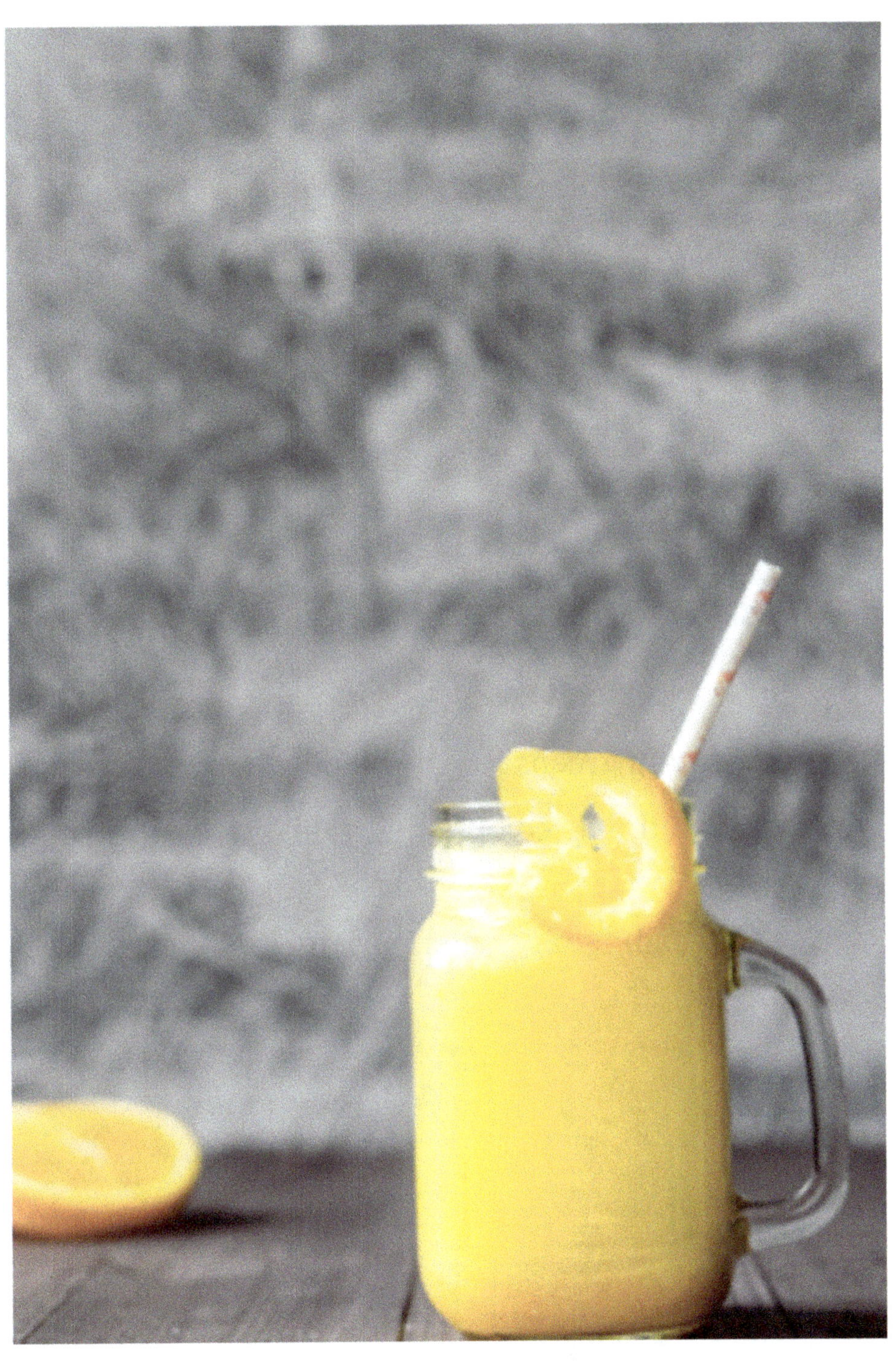

Turnip Smoothie

Ingredients:

Ginger tea, ½ cup

Turnip greens, ½ cup

Date Sugar, 2 teaspoons

Instructions:

1.   Boil ½ cup of water. Add ½ teaspoon of ginger and let it steep for 10-15 minutes.

2.   Strain and let it cool.

3.   Cut turnip greens for the blender.

4.   Blend all ingredients in a high-speed blender until smooth.

5.   Add tea and pulse one more time until mix well.

6.   Enjoy!

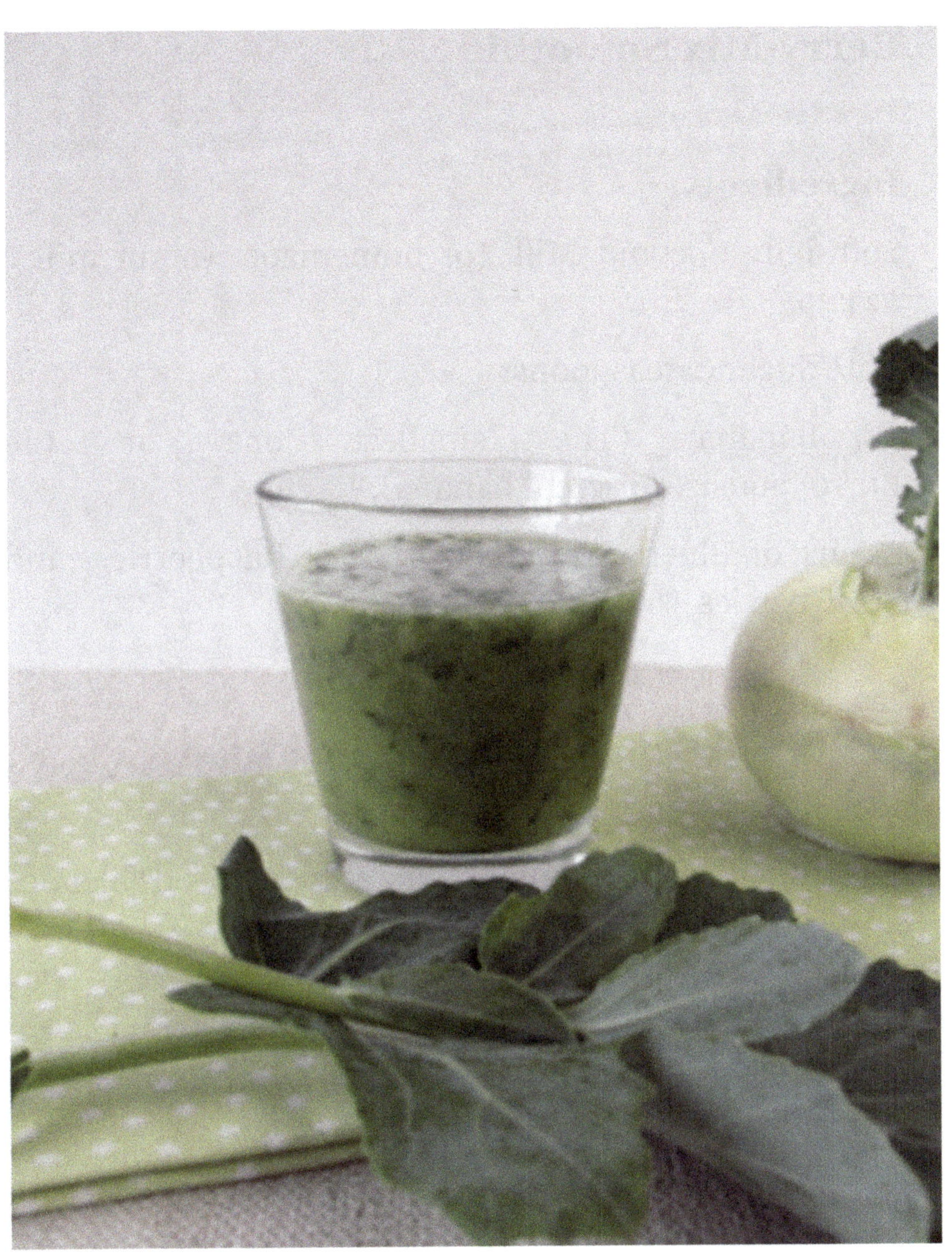

Berry-Mix Smoothie

Ingredients:

Soft Jelly Coconut Milk (or homemade walnut milk), ½ cup

Date Sugar, 2 teaspoons

1 Banana (The smallest one or the Burro/midsize/original banana), ½ cup

A mix of Blueberries, Blackberries, Raspberries, and Strawberries

Instructions:

1. Cut banana for the blender.

2. Blend all ingredients in a high-speed blender until smooth.

3. Enjoy!

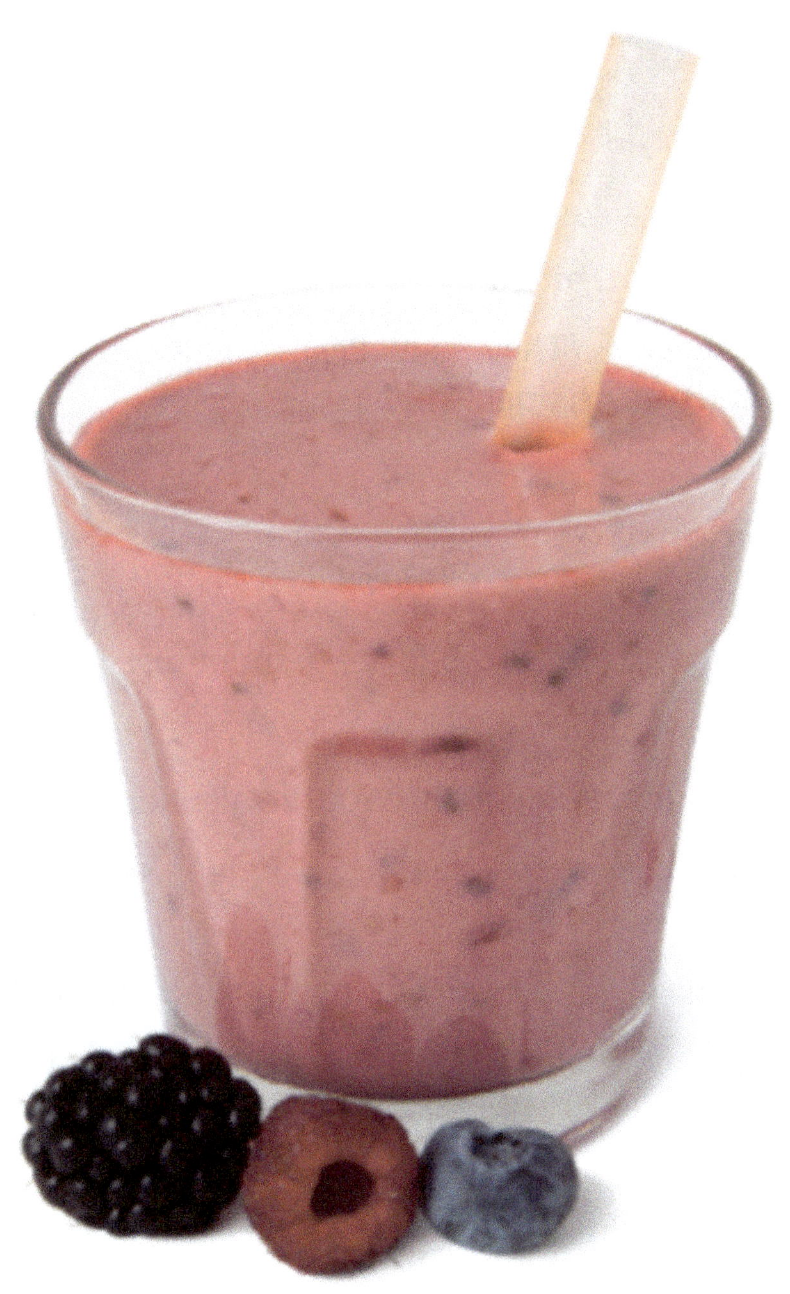

Vitamin-Boost Smoothie

Ingredients:

Chamomile tea, ¼ cup

1 Mango, peeled, pitted

2 Bananas (The smallest one or the Burro/midsize/original banana)

Instructions:

1.   Boil ¼ cup of water. Add ¼ teaspoon of chamomile and let it steep for 10-15 minutes.

2.   Strain and let it cool.

3.   Cut bananas and mango for the blender.

4.   Blend all ingredients in a high-speed blender until smooth.

5.   Add tea and pulse one more time until mix well.

6.   Enjoy!

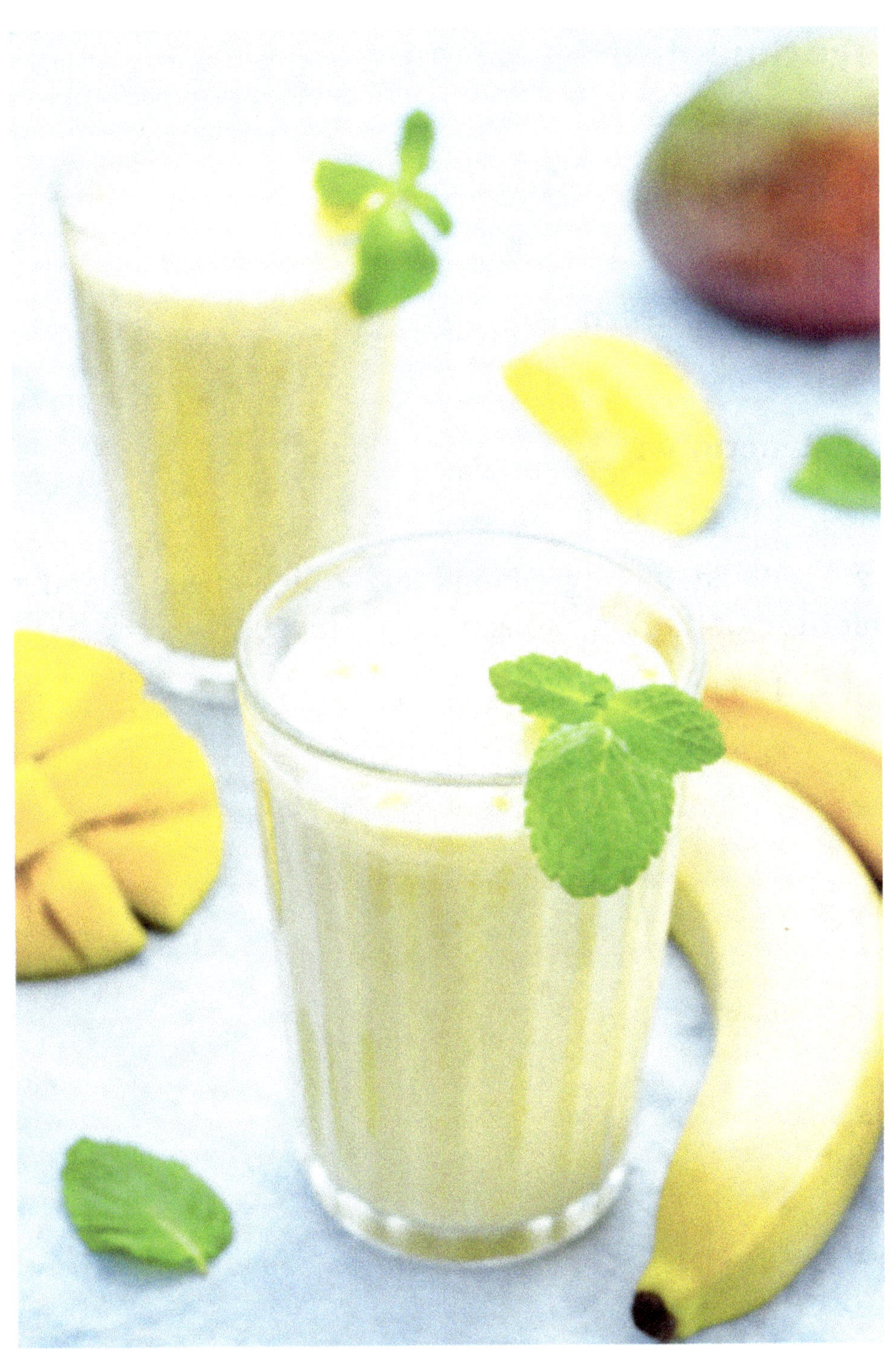

Ice Smoothie

Ingredients:

Ice, ½ cup

1 Mango, peeled, pitted

Instructions:

1.	Cut mango for the blender.

2.	Blend all ingredients in a high-speed blender until smooth. Don't smash ice too much.

3.	Enjoy!

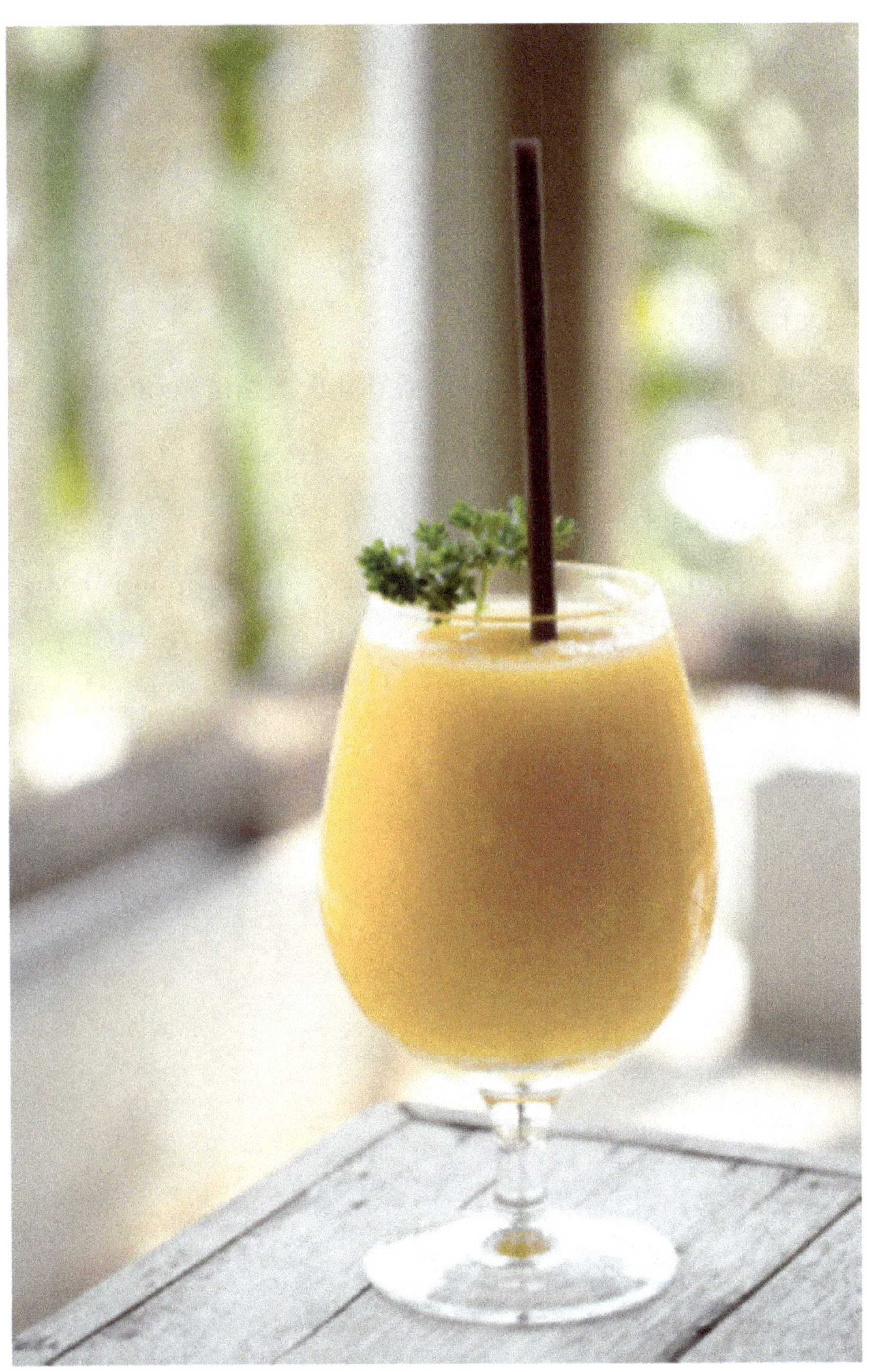

Coconut Smoothie

Ingredients:

Soft Jelly Coconut Water, ½ cup

Date Sugar, 2 teaspoons

Soft Jelly Coconut Pulp, shredded, from 1 coconut

Instructions:

1. Blend all ingredients in a high-speed blender until smooth.

2. Enjoy!

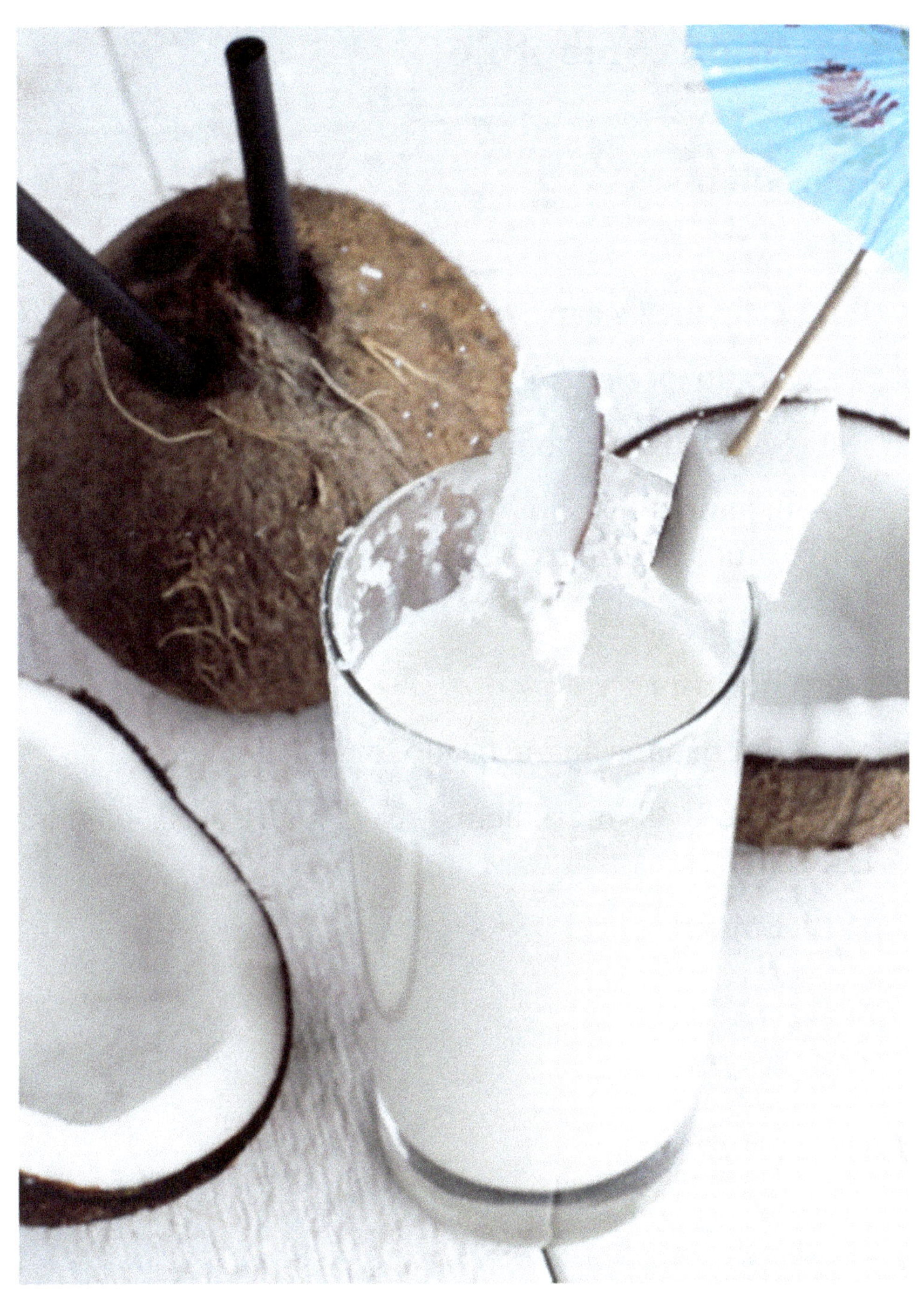

Nutritious Smoothie

Ingredients:

Wild Arugula, ½ cup

½ Avocado, peeled, pitted

Date Sugar, 2 teaspoons

1 Bananas (The smallest one or the Burro/midsize/original banana)

Instructions:

1. Cut banana and avocado for the blender.

2. Blend all ingredients in a high-speed blender until smooth.

3. Enjoy!

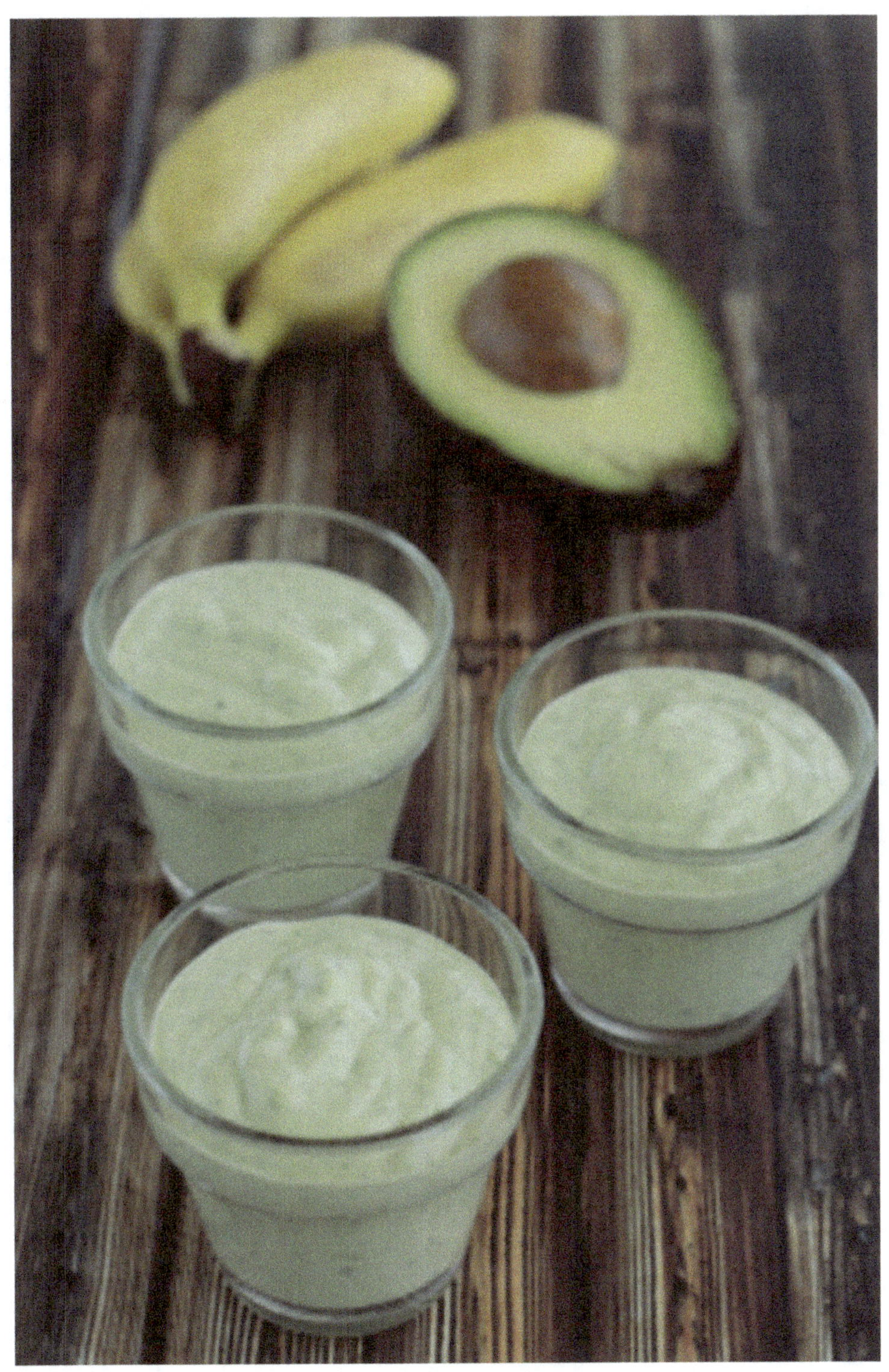

Wakame Smoothie

Ingredients:

2 Bananas (The smallest one or the Burro/midsize/original banana)

Lime juice

1 teaspoon

Chamomile tea, ¼ cup

Wakame (Sea Vegetable), ½ cup

Instructions:

1. Boil ¼ cup of water. Add ½ teaspoon of chamomile and let it steep for 10-15 minutes.

2. Strain and let it cool.

3. Cut bananas for the blender.

4. Blend all ingredients in a high-speed blender until smooth.

5. Enjoy!

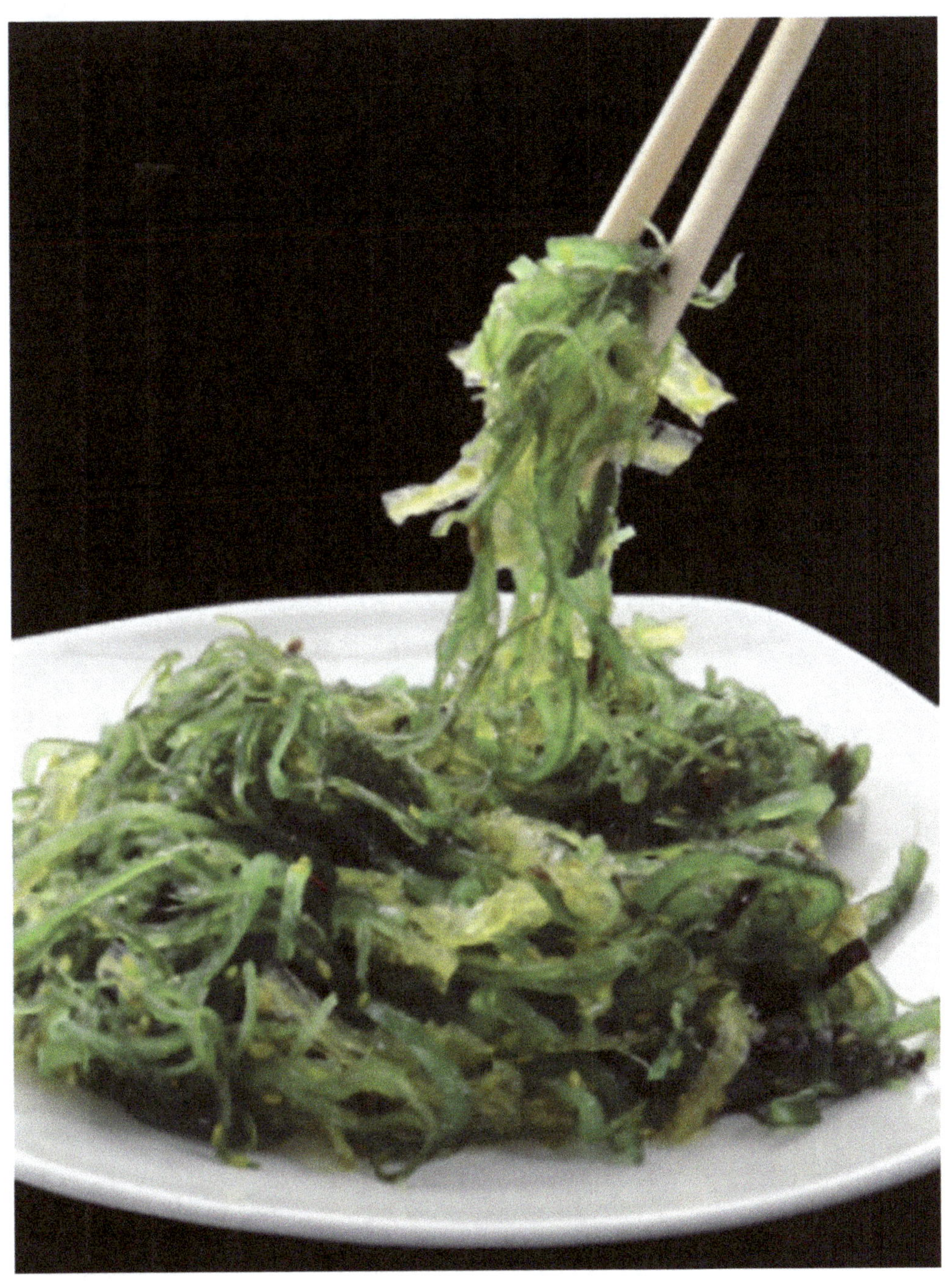

Currant Smoothie

Ingredients:

Soft Jelly Coconut Milk (or homemade walnut milk), ½ cup

Date Sugar, 2 teaspoons

Lime juice, 1 teaspoon

1 Bananas (The smallest one or the Burro/midsize/original banana)

Currants, ½ cup

Instructions:

1. Cut banana for the blender.

2. Blend all ingredients in a high-speed blender until smooth.

3. Enjoy!

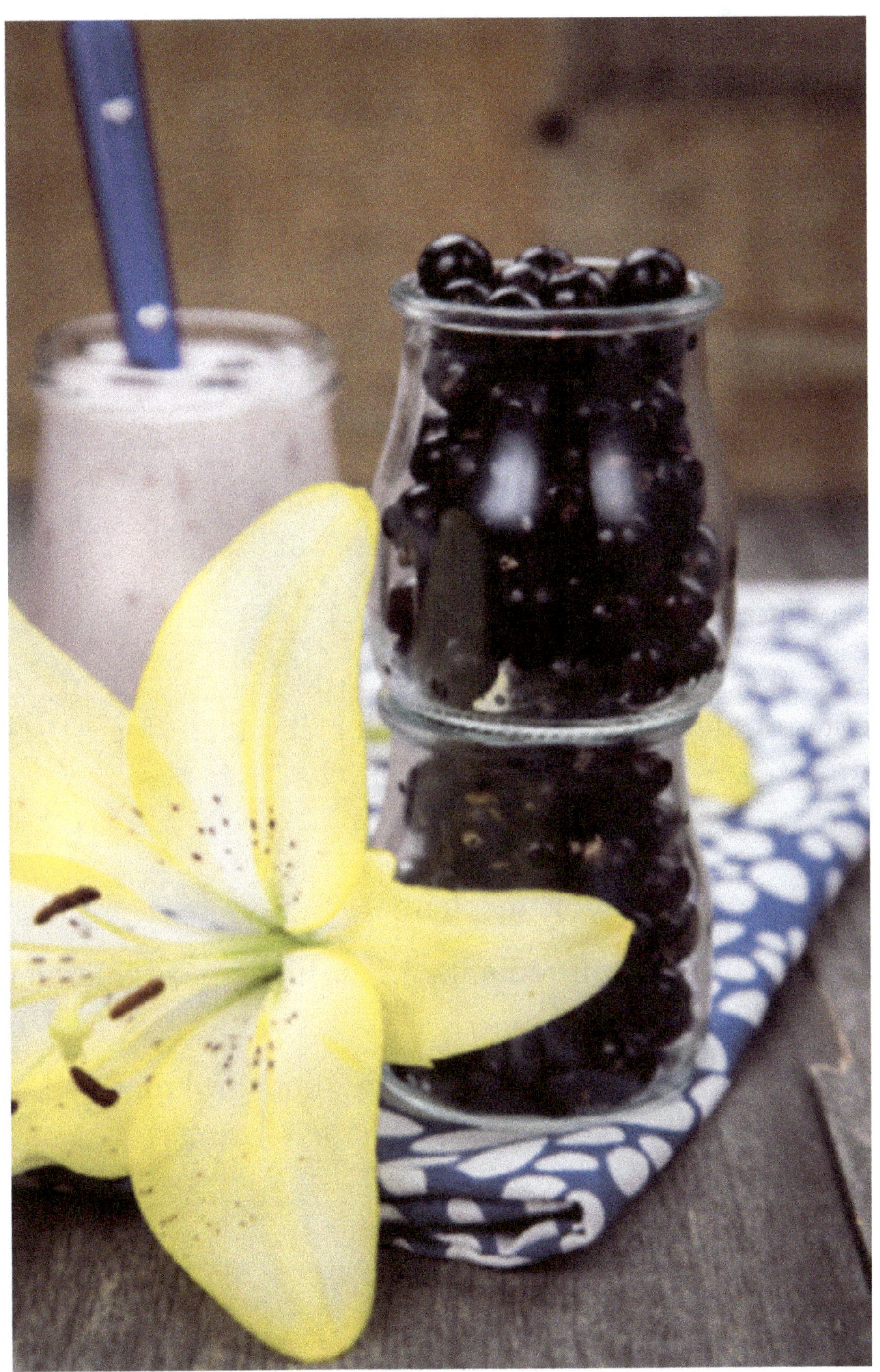

Plum Smoothie

Ingredients:

Chamomile or Burdock tea, ¼ cup

5, Plums, pitted

Date Sugar, 2 teaspoons

1 Bananas (The smallest one or the Burro/midsize/original banana)

Instructions:

1. Boil ¼ cup of water. Add ¼ teaspoon of chamomile or burdock and let it steep for 10-15 minutes.

2. Strain and let it cool.

3. Cut banana for the blender.

4. Blend all ingredients in a high-speed blender until smooth.

5. Add tea and pulse one more time until mix well.

6. Enjoy!

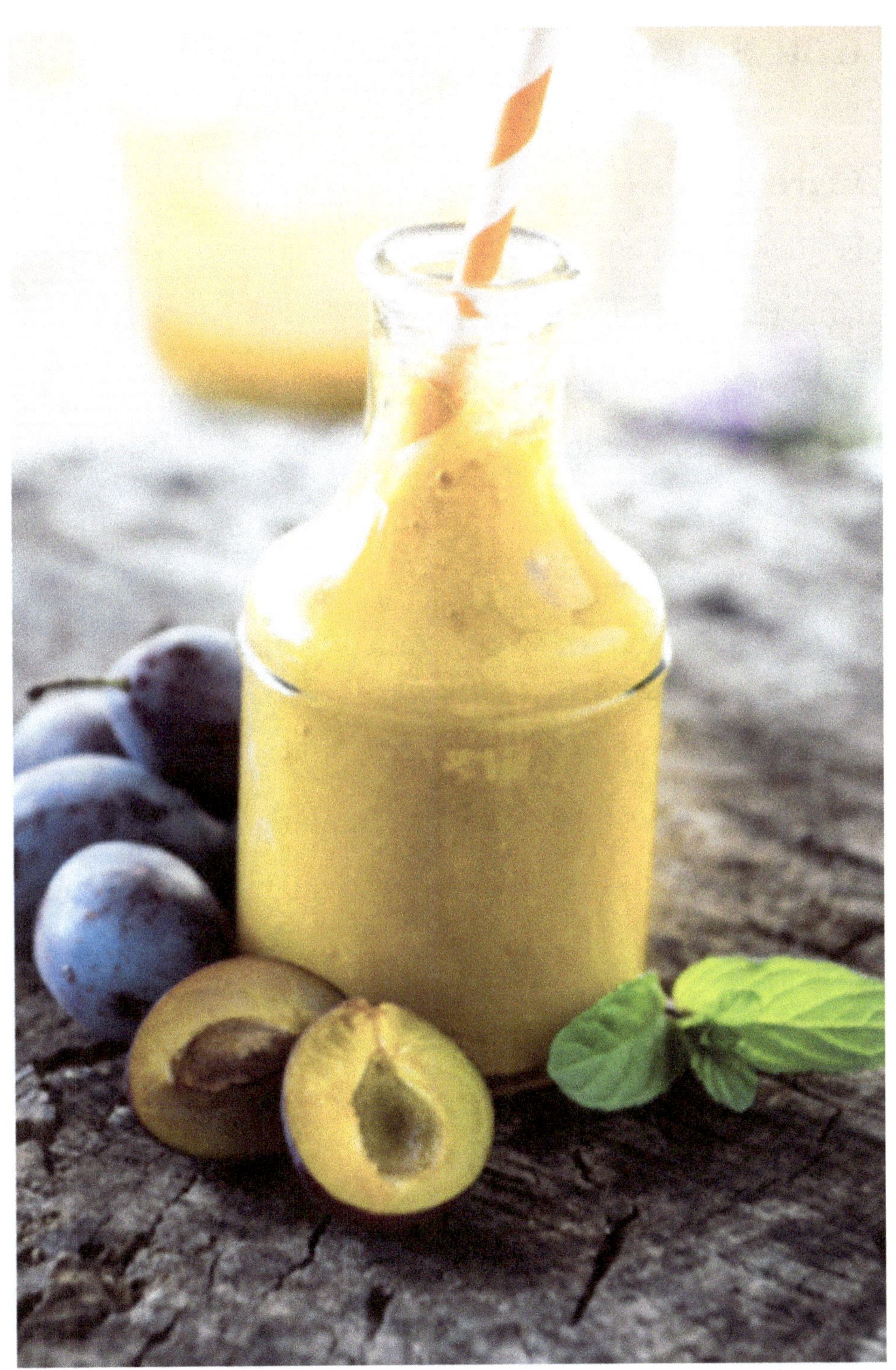

Izote Smoothie

Ingredients:

Fennel tea, ¼ cup

Izote (Cactus leaf), about ½ cup

Date Sugar, 2 teaspoons

Raspberries, ¼ cup

Instructions:

1.   Boil ¼ cup of water. Add ¼ teaspoon of fennel and let it steep for 10-15 minutes.

2.   Strain and let it cool.

3.   Cut cactus leaves for the blender.

4.   Blend all ingredients in a high-speed blender until smooth.

5.   Add tea and pulse one more time until mix well.

6.   Enjoy!

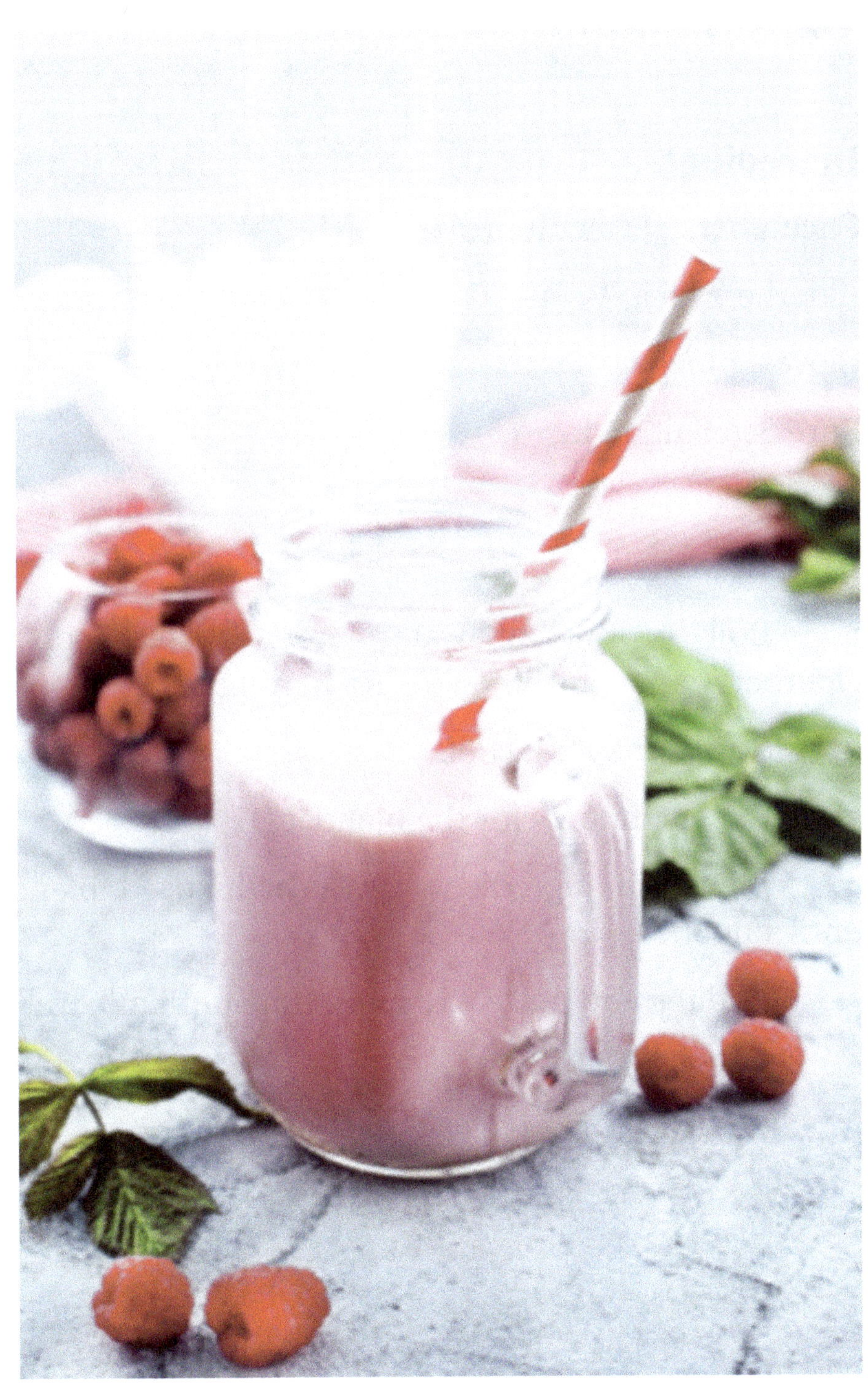

Tonic Smoothie

Ingredients:

Cucumbers, 3 (medium size)

Elderberry tea, ¼ cup,

Cloves, pinch

Pure Sea Salt, to taste

Instructions:

1.   Boil ¼ cup of water. Add ¼ teaspoon of elderberry and let it steep for 10-15 minutes.

2.   Strain and let it cool.

3.   Cut cucumbers for the blender.

4.   Blend all ingredients in a high-speed blender until smooth.

5.   Add tea and pulse one more time until mix well.

6.   Enjoy!

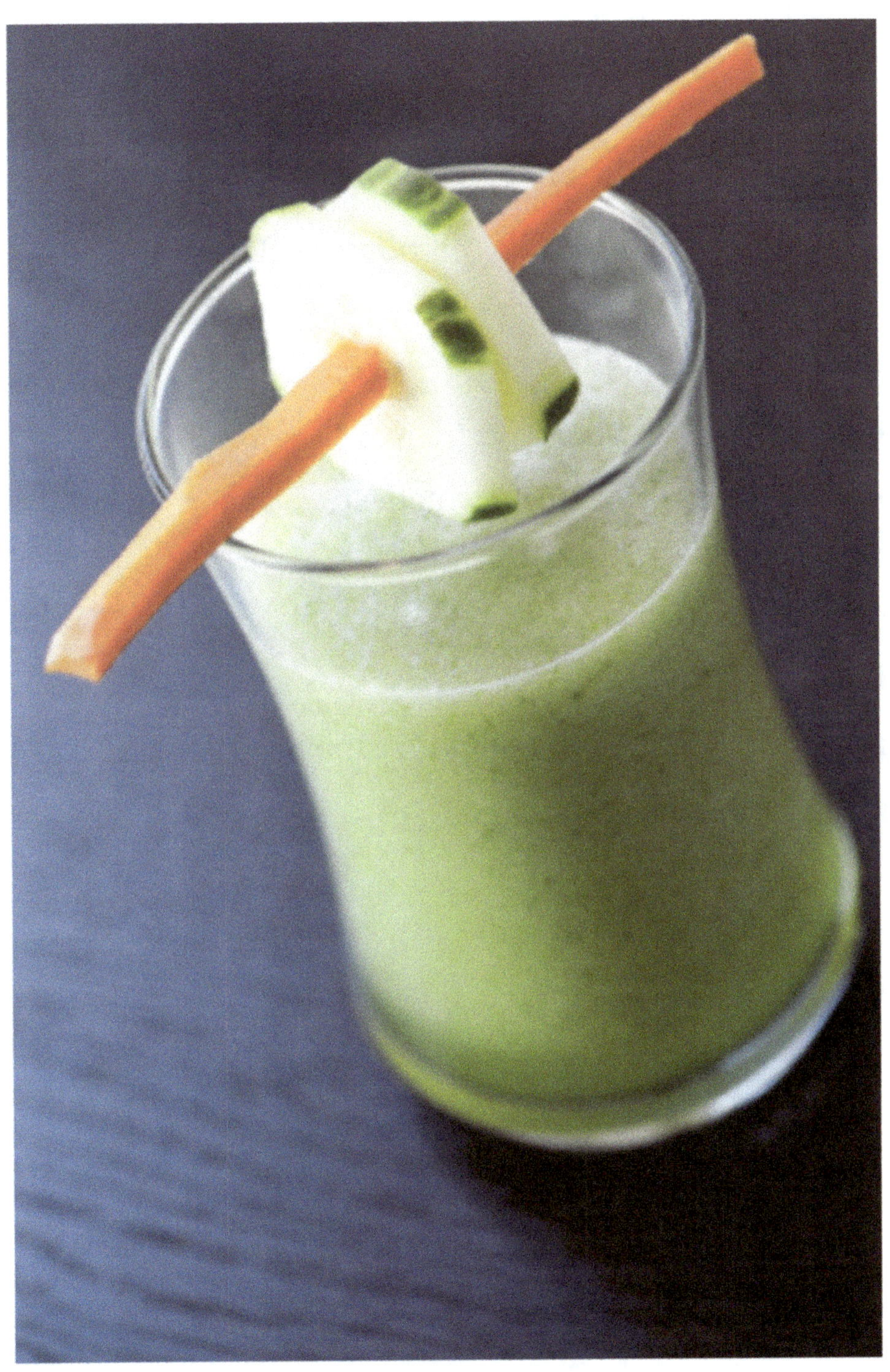

Tender Mango Smoothie

Ingredients:

Soft Jelly Coconut Milk (or homemade walnut milk), ½ cup

1 Mango, peeled, pitted

Blueberries, ¼ cup

1 Bananas (The smallest one or the Burro/midsize/original banana)

Instructions:

1. Cut banana and mango for the blender.

2. Blend all ingredients in a high-speed blender until smooth.

3. Pour the mixture into a nut milk bag.

4. Enjoy!

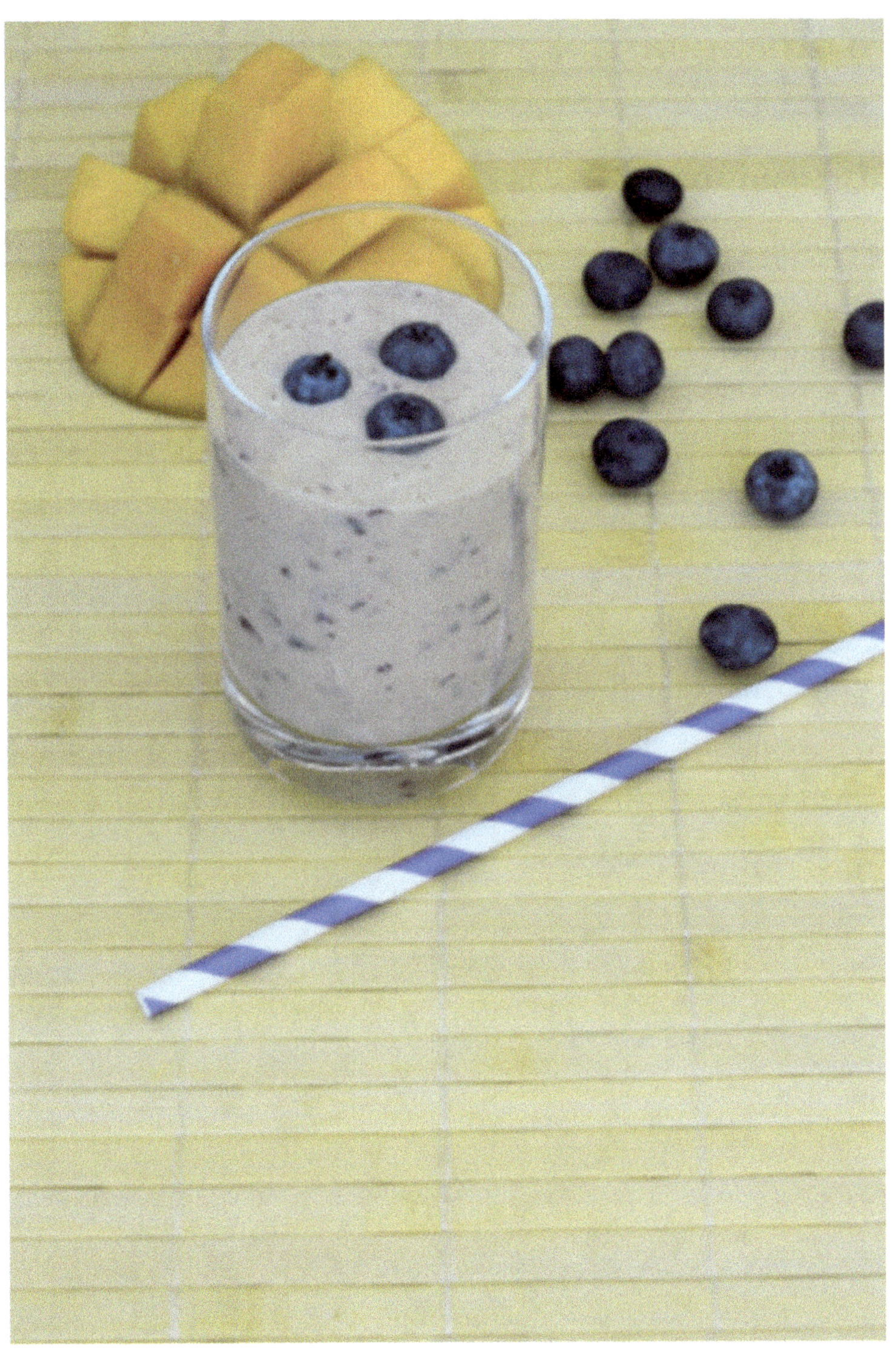

Nutty Squash Smoothie

Ingredients:

Squash, ½ cup

Soft Jelly Coconut Milk (or homemade walnut milk), ¼ cup

Date Sugar, 2 teaspoons

Brazil Nuts or Walnuts, ¼ cup

Instructions:

1.   Cut squash for the blender.

2.   Blend all ingredients in a high-speed blender until smooth.

3.   Enjoy!

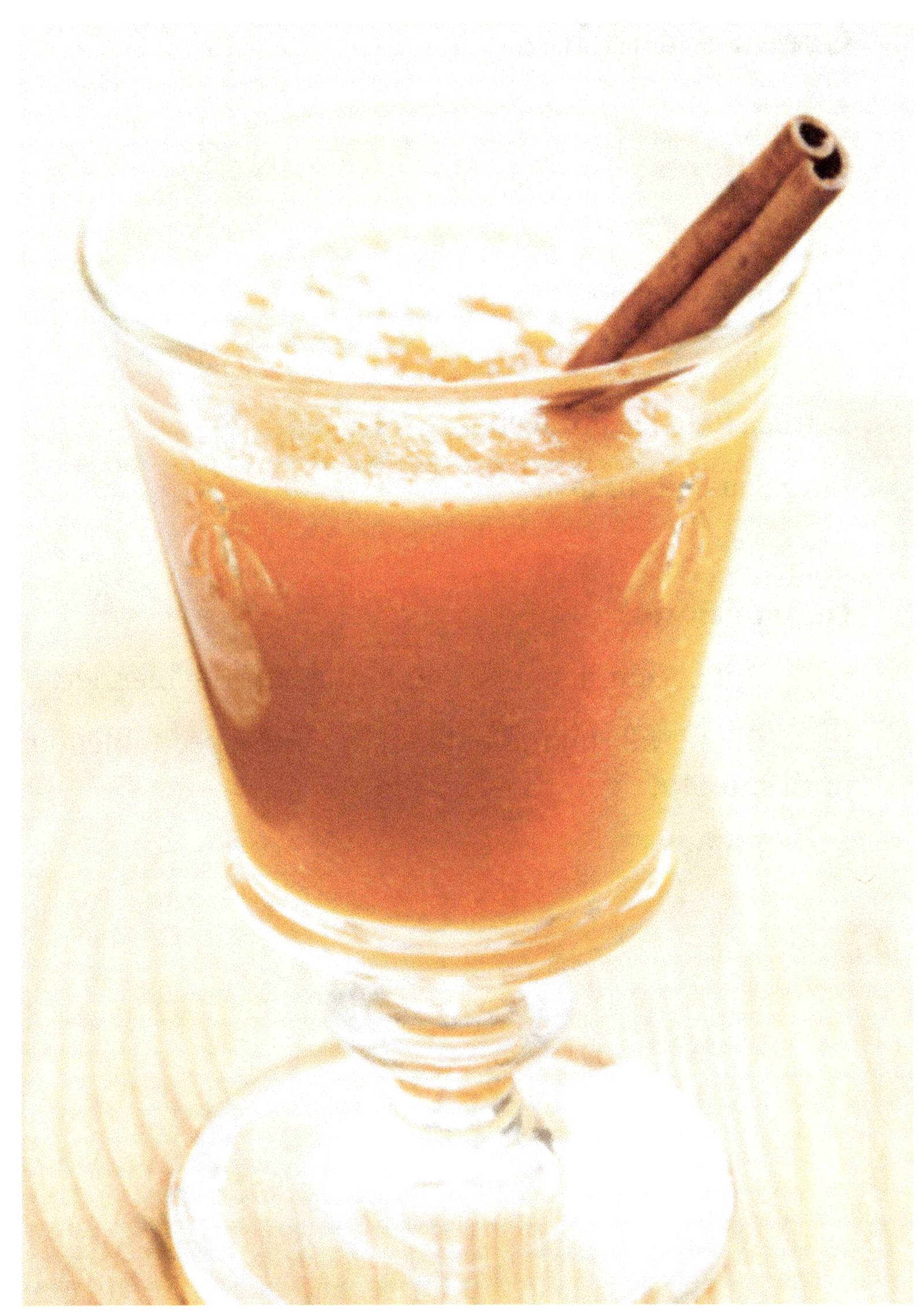

Green Smoothie

Ingredients:

Zucchini, ½ (medium size)

1 Apple

Lettuce (All, except Iceberg), 2 leaves

Pure Sea Salt, to taste

Instructions:

1.	Cut zucchini, apple, and lettuce for the blender.

2.	Blend all ingredients in a high-speed blender until smooth.

3.	Enjoy!

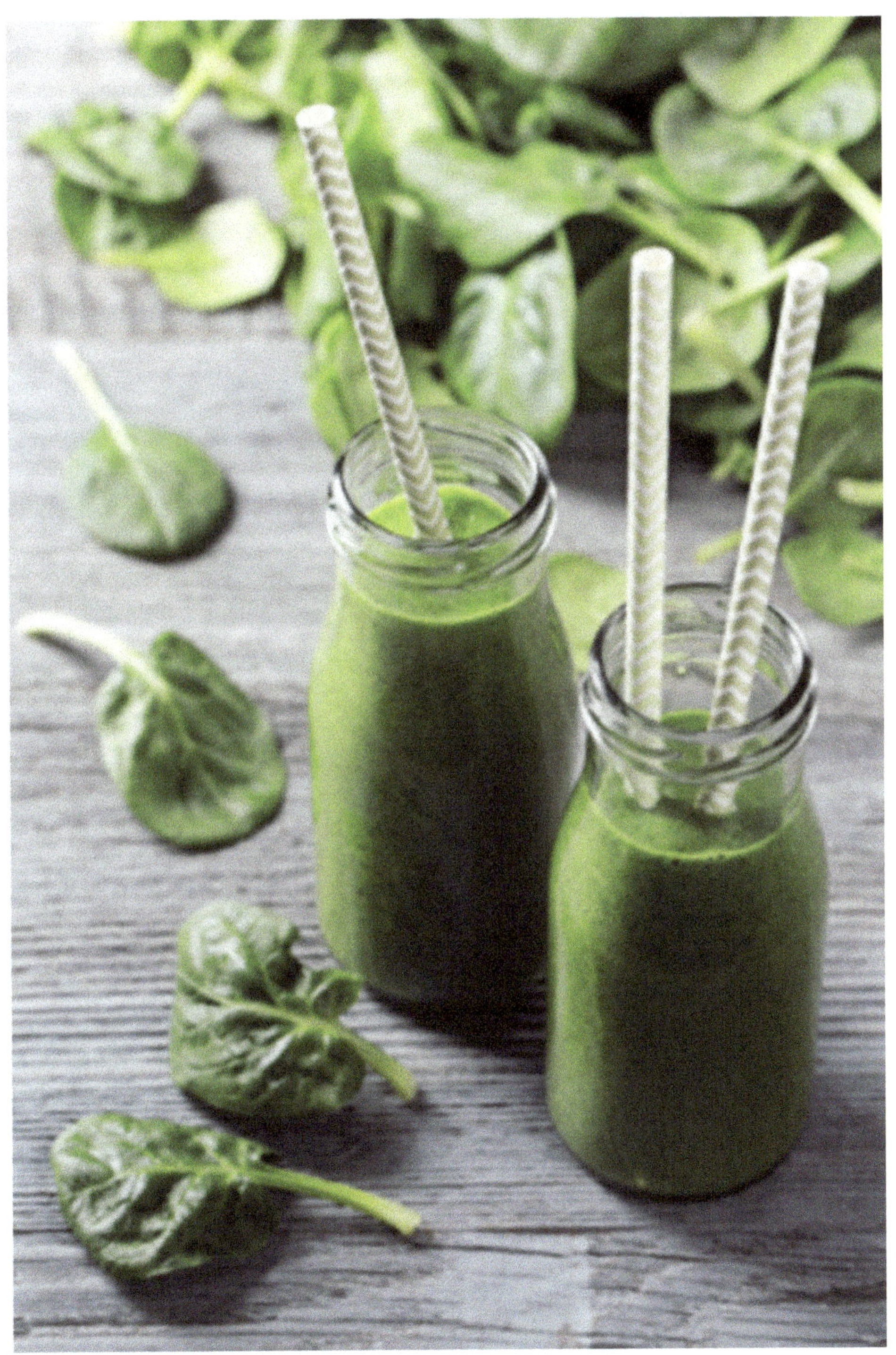

Sweet Mix Smoothie

Ingredients:

Soft Jelly Coconut Milk (or homemade walnut milk), ½ cup

Date Sugar, 2 teaspoons

Blueberries, ¼ cup

Strawberries, ¼ cup

1 Figs, peeled

Instructions:

1. Cut figs for the blender.

2. Blend all ingredients in a high-speed blender until smooth.

3. Enjoy!

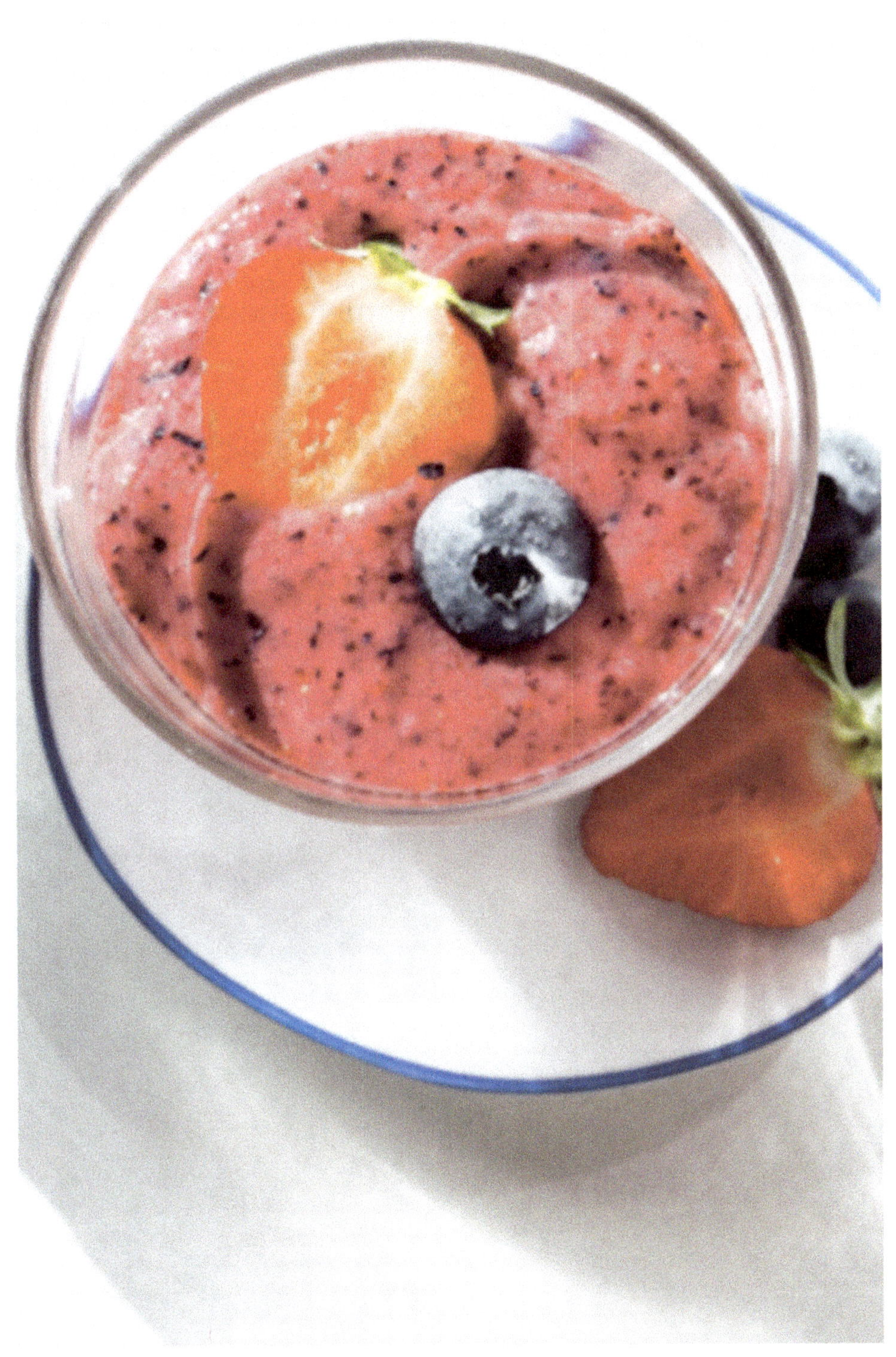

Papaya Smoothie

Ingredients:

Soft Jelly Coconut Milk (or homemade walnut milk), ½ cup

Papayas, 4 oz (113 g)

Ginger, grated, ¼ teaspoons

Instructions:

1.   Cut papaya for the blender.

2.   Blend all ingredients in a high-speed blender until smooth.

3.   Enjoy!

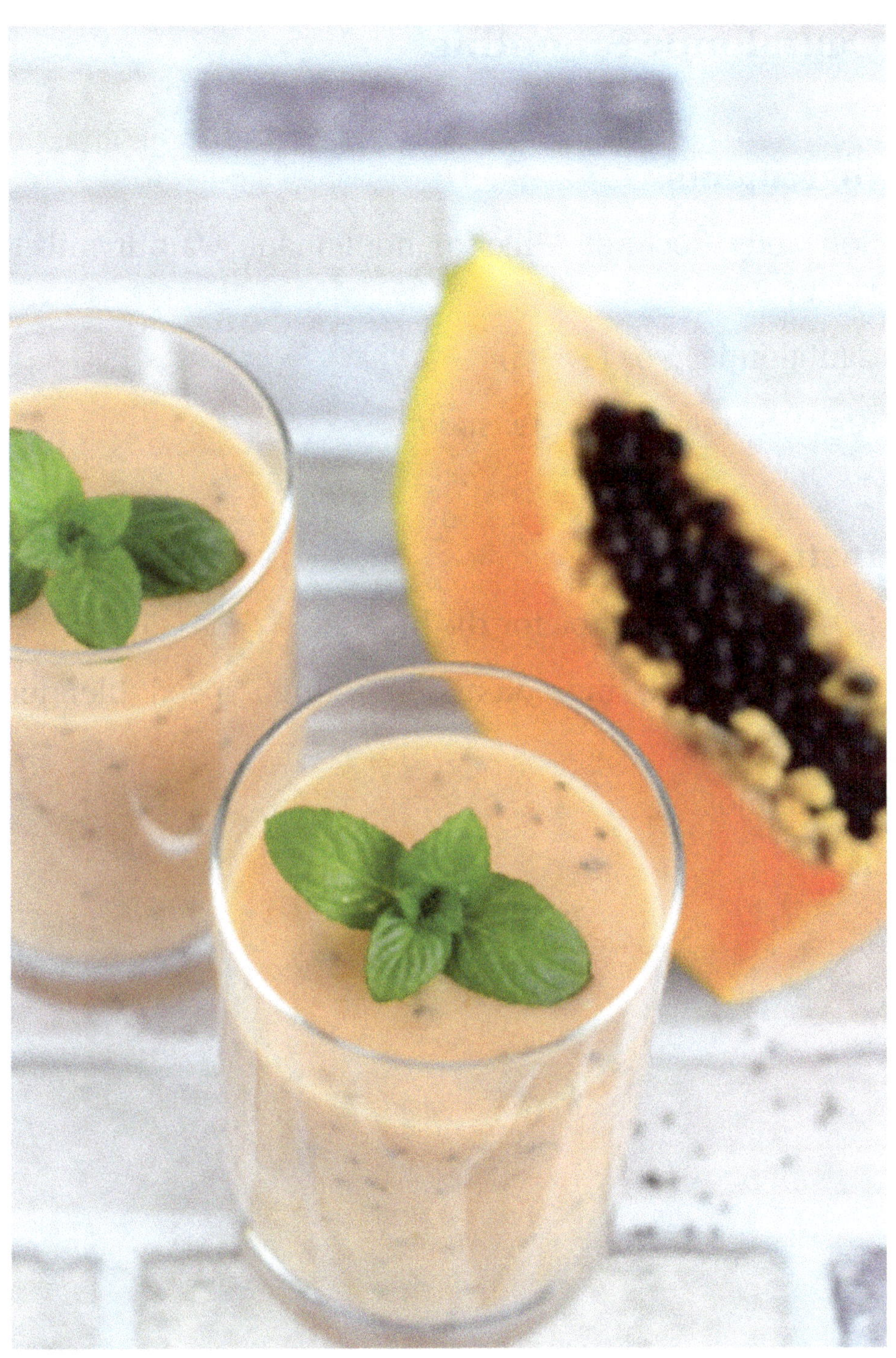

Cantaloupe Smoothie

Ingredients:

Soft Jelly Coconut Milk (or homemade walnut milk), ¼ cup

Cantaloupe, 6 oz (170 g)

Raw Sesame Seeds, 1 teaspoon

Instructions:

1.	Cut cantaloupe for the blender.

2.	Blend all ingredients in a high-speed blender until smooth.

3.	Enjoy!

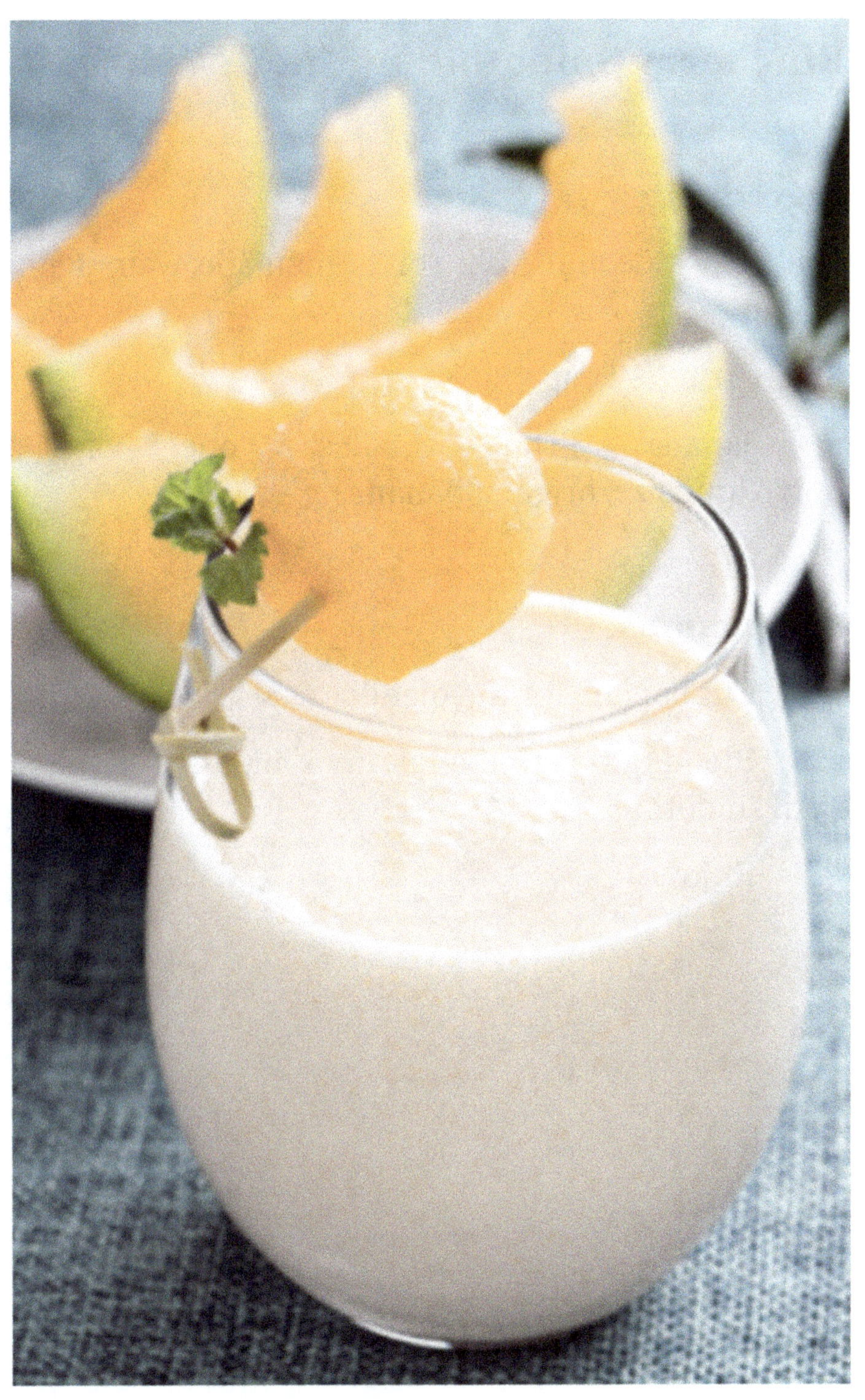

Blueberry Smoothie

Ingredients:

Soft Jelly Coconut Milk (or homemade walnut milk), ½ cup

Blueberries, ½ cup

1 Banana (The smallest one or the Burro/midsize/original banana)

Instructions:

1. Cut banana for the blender.

2. Blend all ingredients in a high-speed blender until smooth.

3. Enjoy!

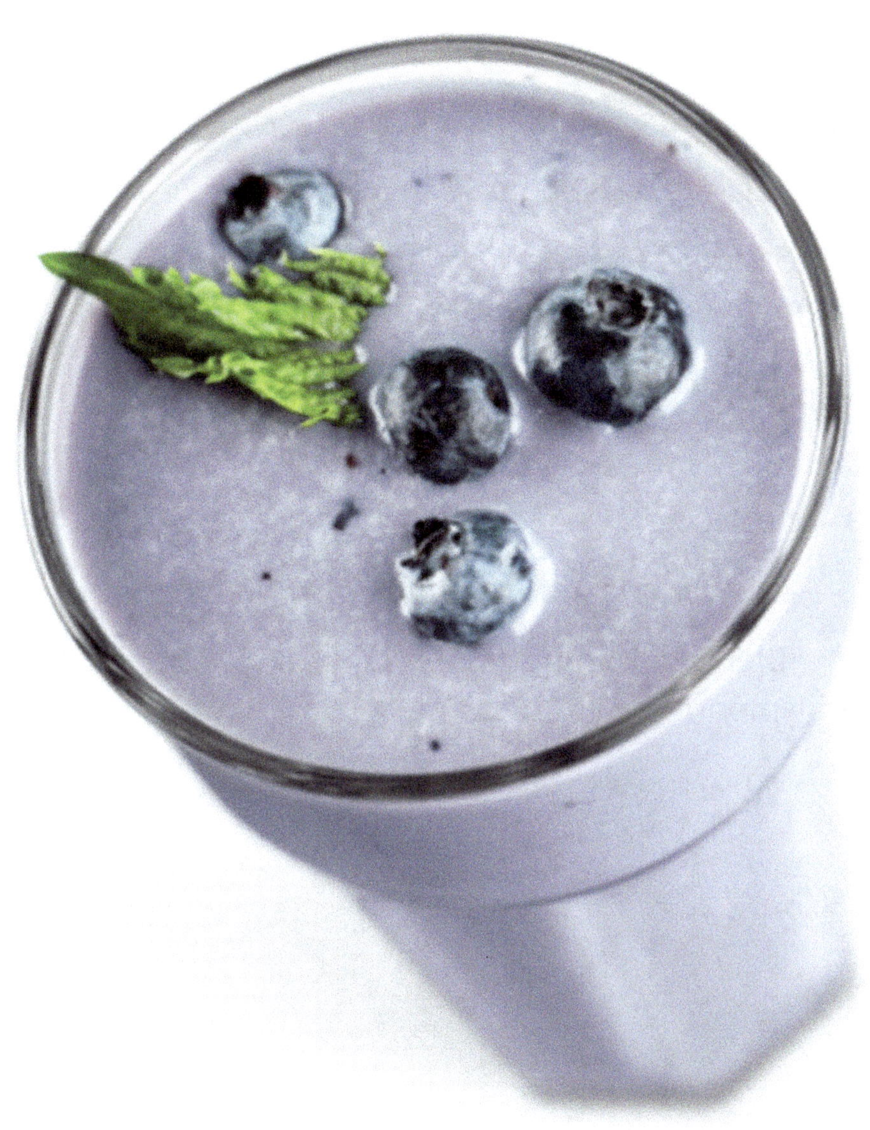

Pear Smoothie

Ingredients:

Date Sugar, 2 teaspoons

1 Banana (The smallest one or the Burro/midsize/original banana)

3 Pears, pitted

Instructions:

1. Cut banana and pears for the blender.

2. Blend all ingredients in a high-speed blender until smooth.

3. Enjoy!

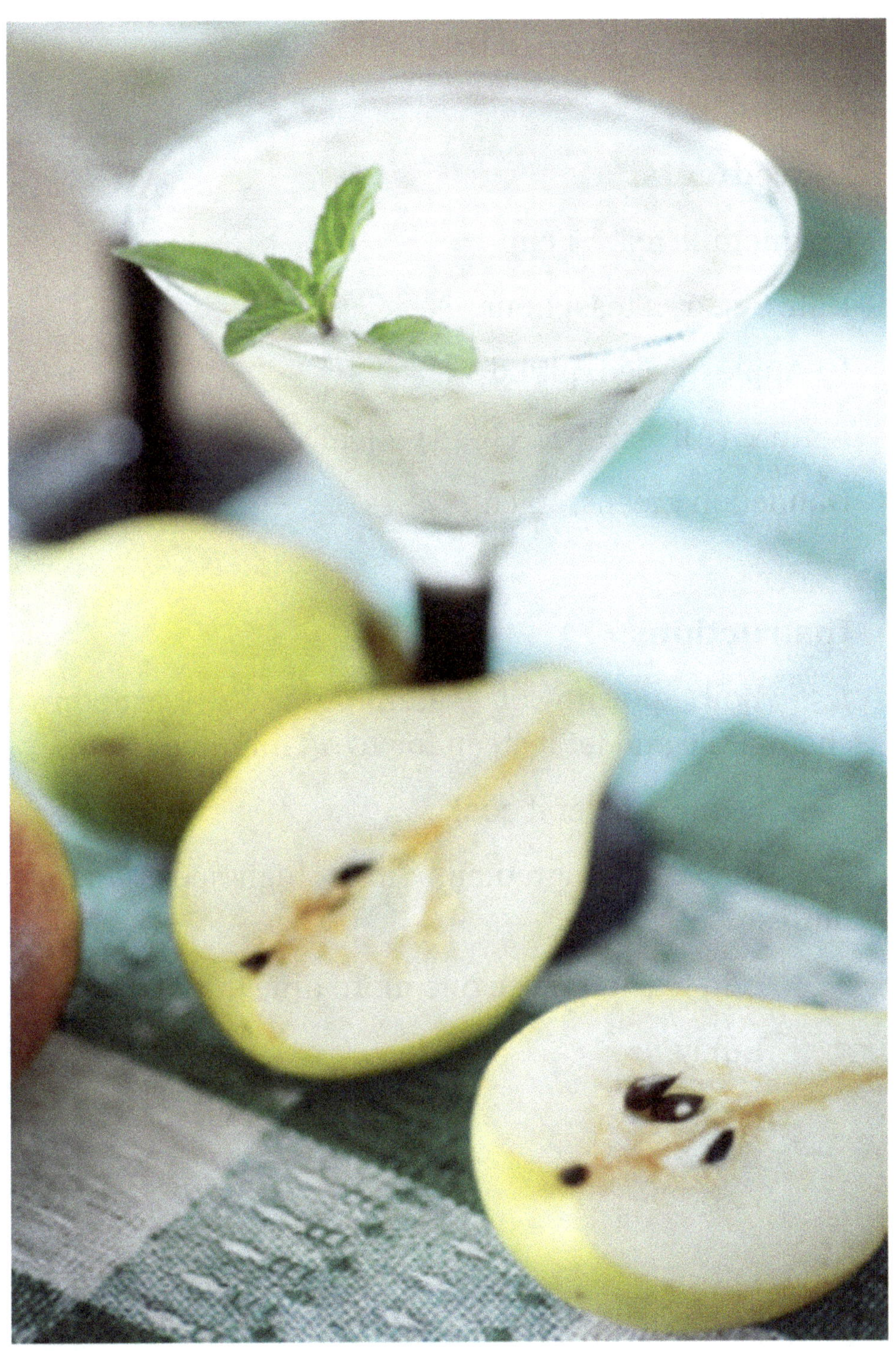

Dandelion Smoothie

Ingredients:

Chamomile tea, ¼ cup

Date Sugar, 2 teaspoons

½ Apple, peeled, pitted

Lettuce (All, except Iceberg), 1 leaf

Dandelion greens, ½ cup

Instructions:

1. Boil ¼ cup of water. Add ½ teaspoon of chamomile and let it steep for 10-15 minutes.

2. Strain and let it cool.

3. Blend all ingredients in a high-speed blender until smooth.

4. Add tea and pulse one more time until mix well.

5. Enjoy!

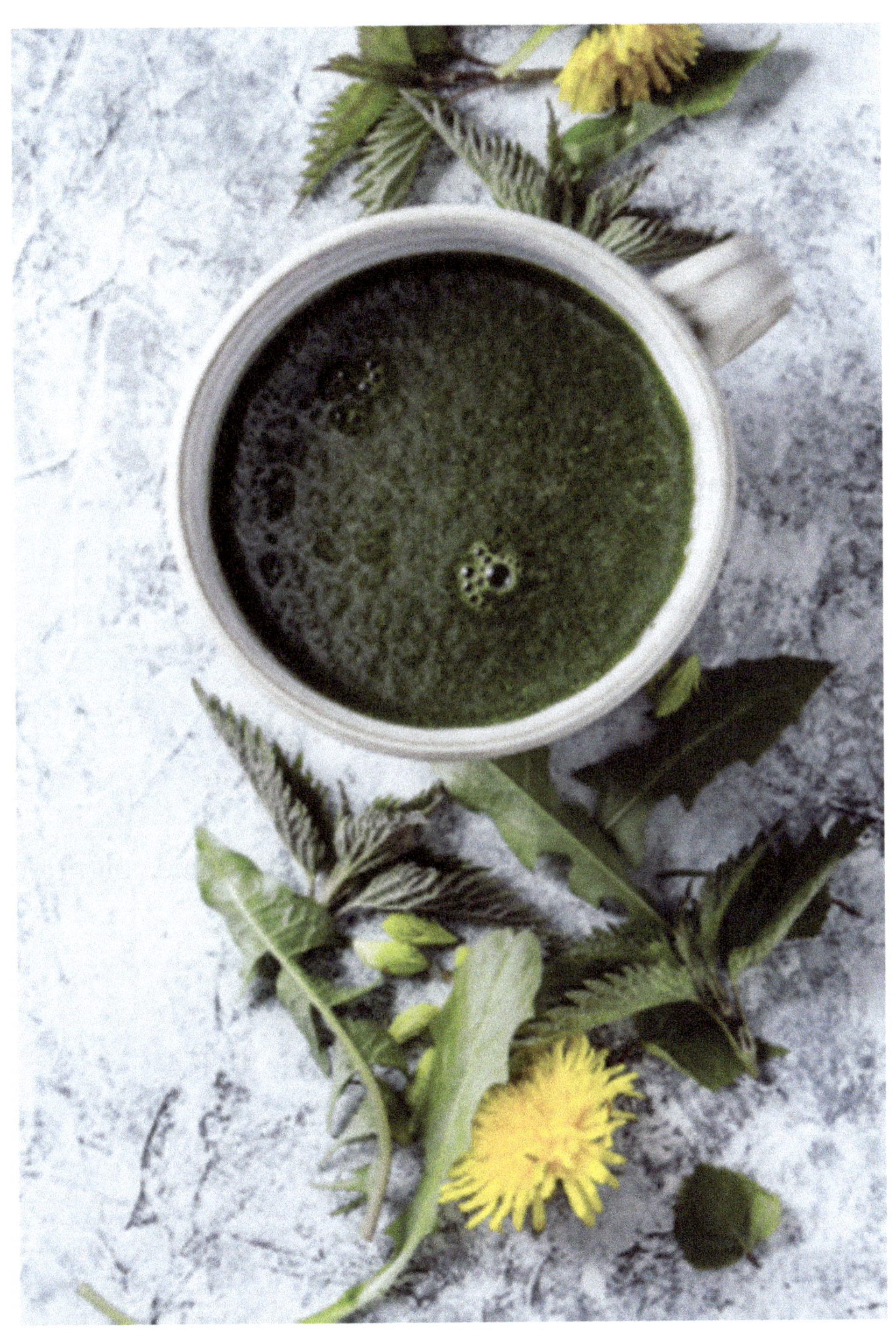

Banana and Quinoa Smoothie

Ingredients:

Soft Jelly Coconut Milk (or homemade walnut milk), ½ cup

Date Sugar, 2 teaspoons

Quinoa, cooked, ¼ cup

Brazil Nuts or Walnuts, ¼ cup

1 Bananas (The smallest one or the Burro/midsize/original banana)

Instructions:

1. Cut banana for the blender.

2. Blend all ingredients in a high-speed blender until smooth.

3. Enjoy!

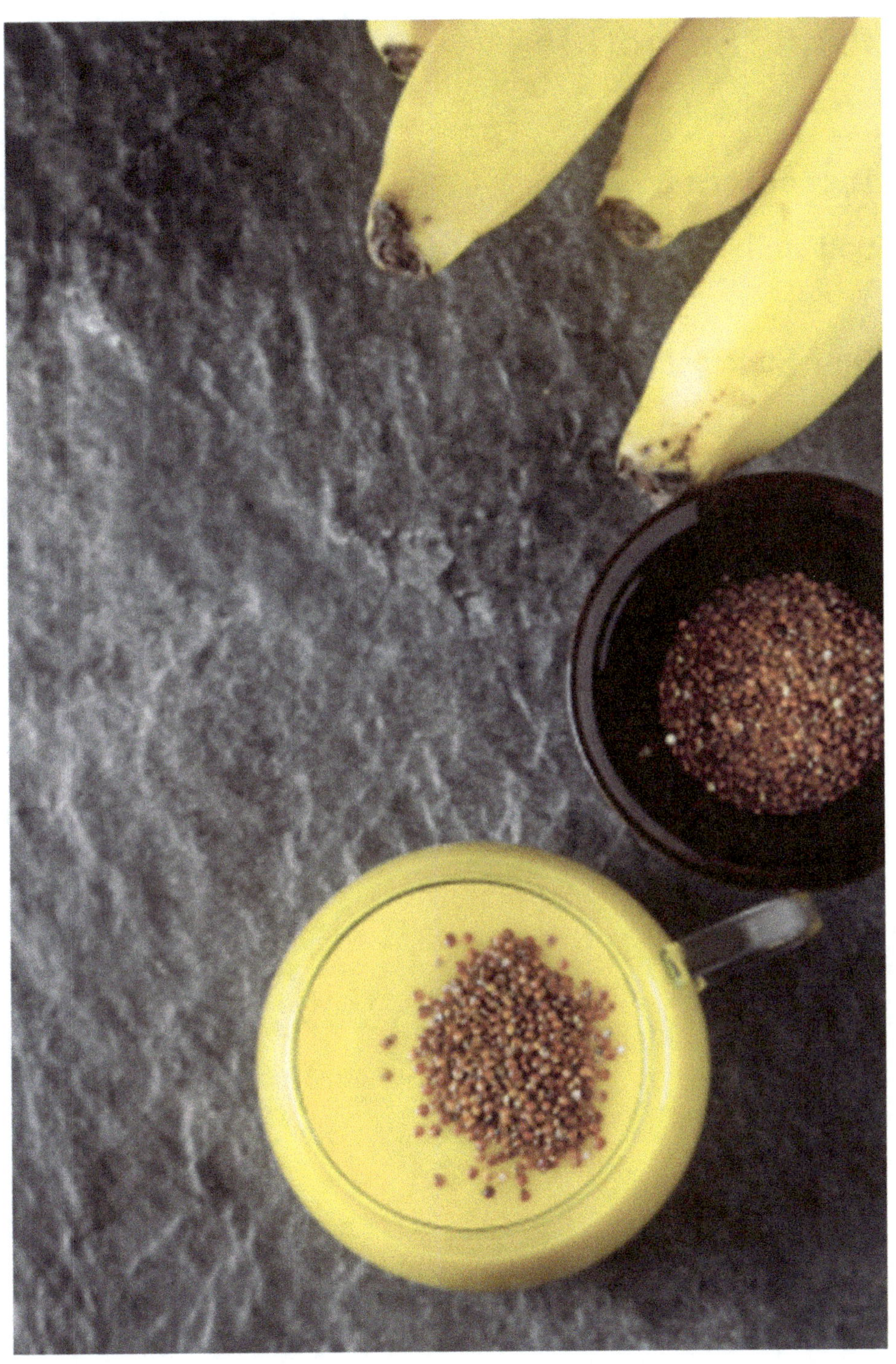

Prune Smoothie

Ingredients:

Soft Jelly Coconut Milk (or homemade walnut milk), ½ cup

Date Sugar, 2 teaspoons

Prunes, ¼ cup

1 Bananas (The smallest one or the Burro/midsize/original banana)

Instructions:

1. Cut banana for the blender.

2. Blend all ingredients in a high-speed blender until smooth.

3. Enjoy!

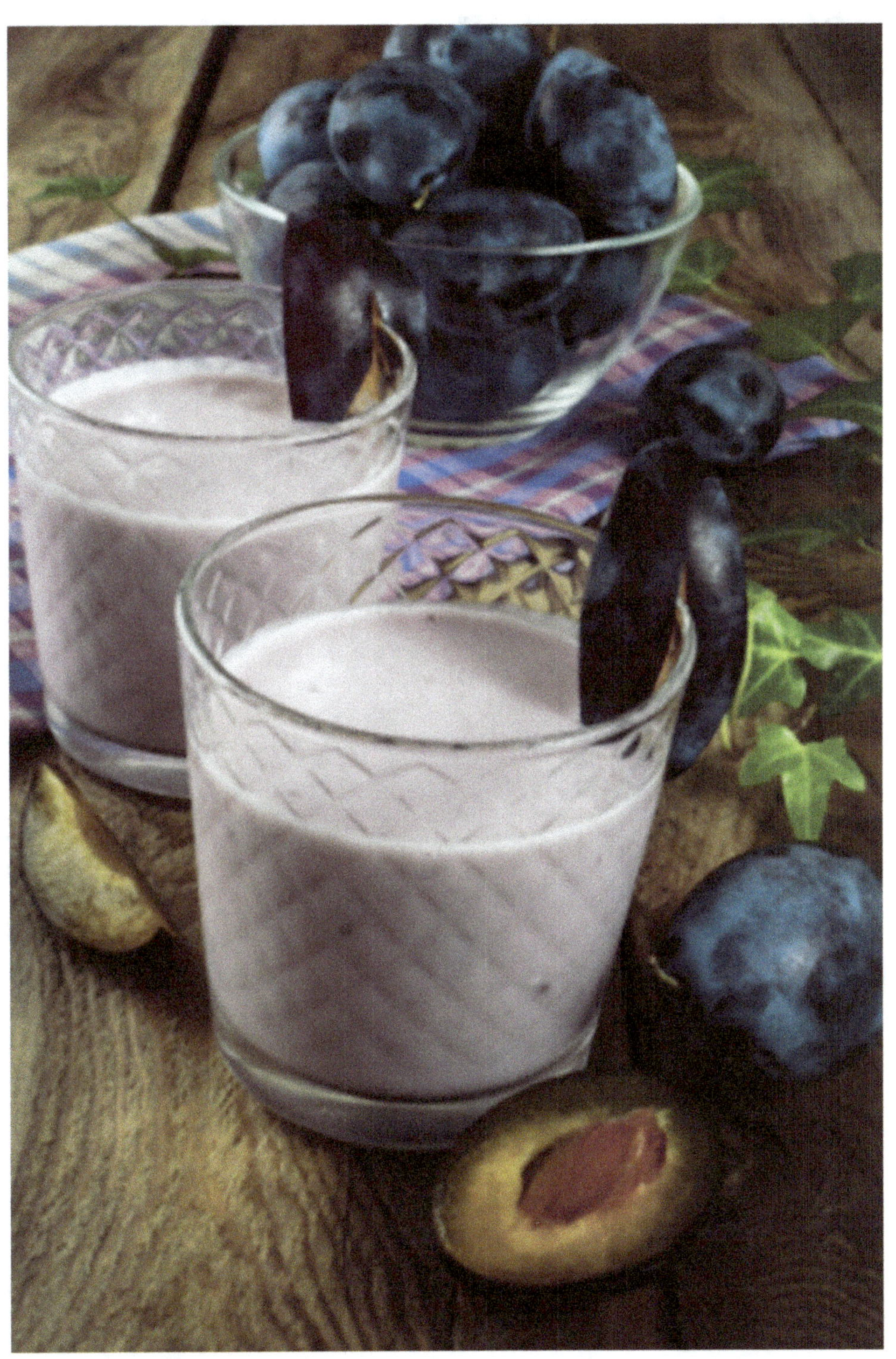

Strawberry Smoothie

Ingredients:

Ginger tea, ¼ cup

Date Sugar, 2 teaspoons

Strawberries, ¾ cup

Instructions:

1.   Boil ¼ cup of water. Add ½ teaspoon of ginger and let it steep for 10-15 minutes.

2.   Strain and let it cool.

3.   Blend all ingredients in a high-speed blender until smooth.

4.   Add tea and pulse one more time until mix well.

5.   Enjoy!

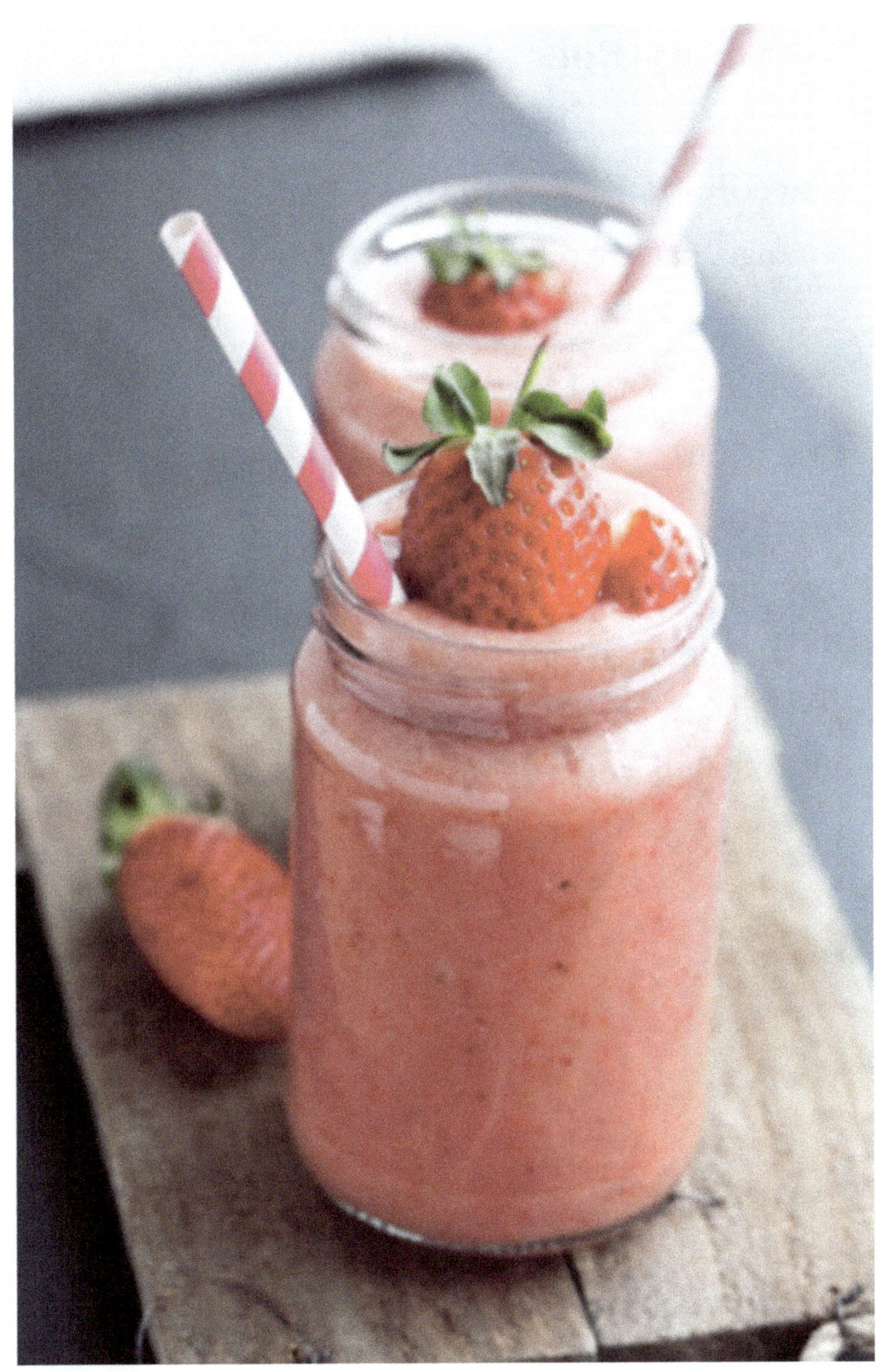

Immunity-Boost Smoothie

Ingredients:

1 Mango, peeled, pitted

Strawberries, ½ cup

Olive Oil (Do not cook)

1 teaspoon

Instructions:

1.   Cut mango for the blender.

2.   Blend all ingredients in a high-speed blender until smooth.

3.   Enjoy!

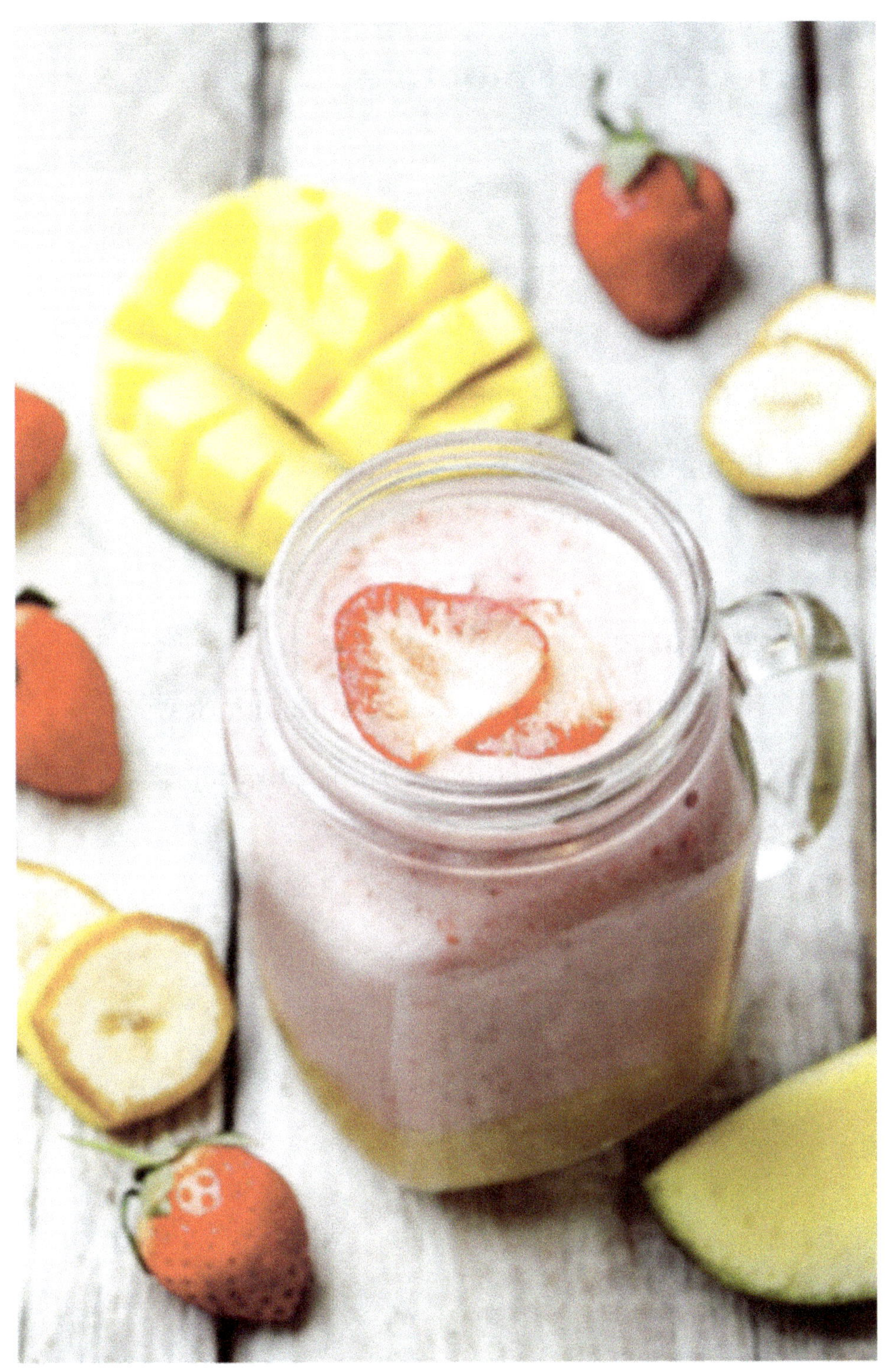

Perfect Apple Smoothie

Ingredients:

Strawberries, ½ cup

2 Apples

Date Sugar, 2 teaspoons

1 Bananas (The smallest one or the Burro/midsize/original banana)

Instructions:

1. Cut banana and apples for the blender.

2. Blend all ingredients in a high-speed blender until smooth.

3. Enjoy!

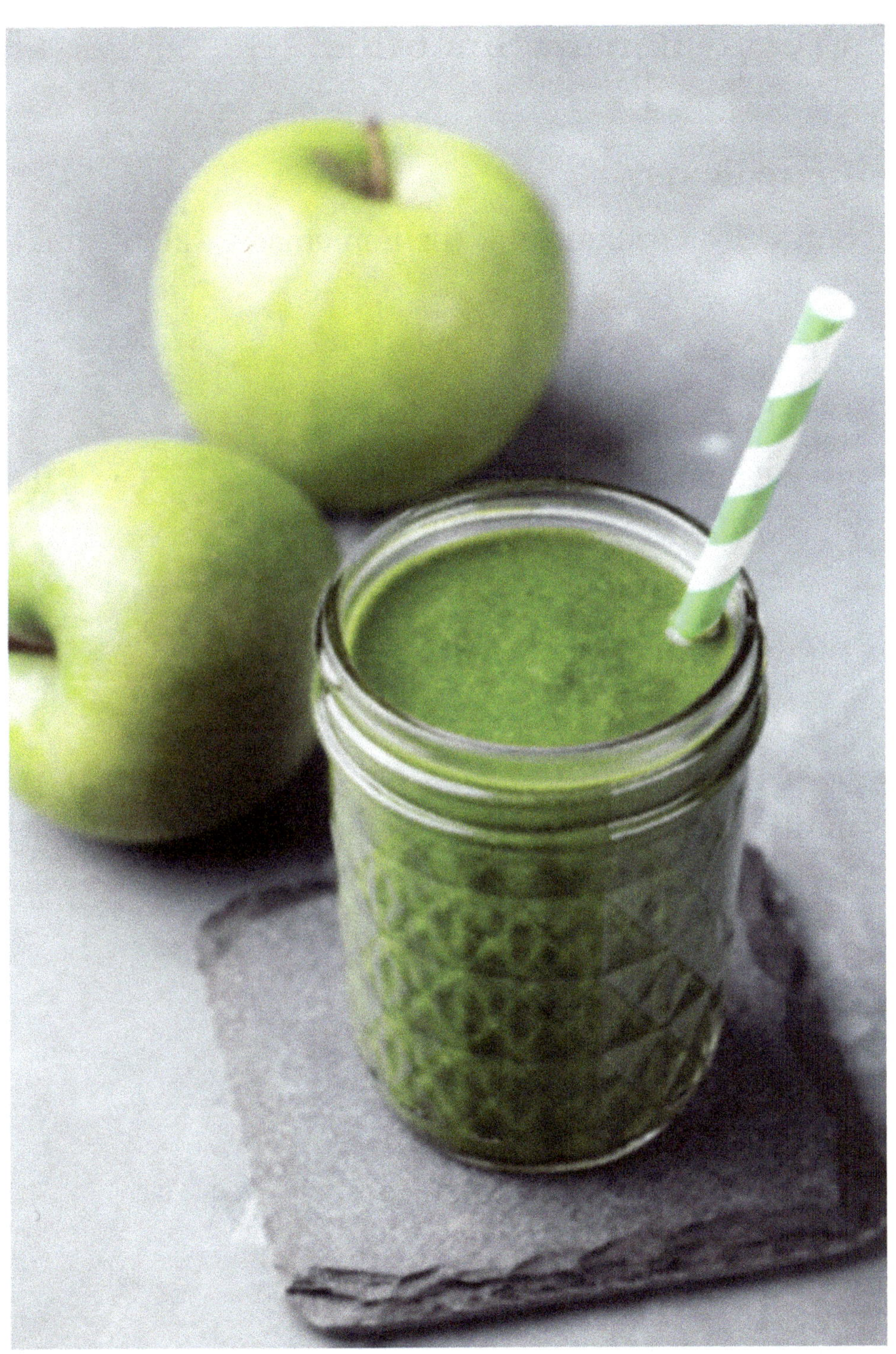

Creamy Banana Smoothie

Ingredients:

Soft Jelly Coconut Milk (or homemade walnut milk), ½ cup

Brazil Nuts or Walnuts, ¼ cup

Date Sugar, 2 teaspoons

3 Bananas (The smallest one or the Burro/midsize/original banana)

Instructions:

1.   Cut bananas for the blender.

2.   Blend all ingredients in a high-speed blender until creamy.

3.   Enjoy!

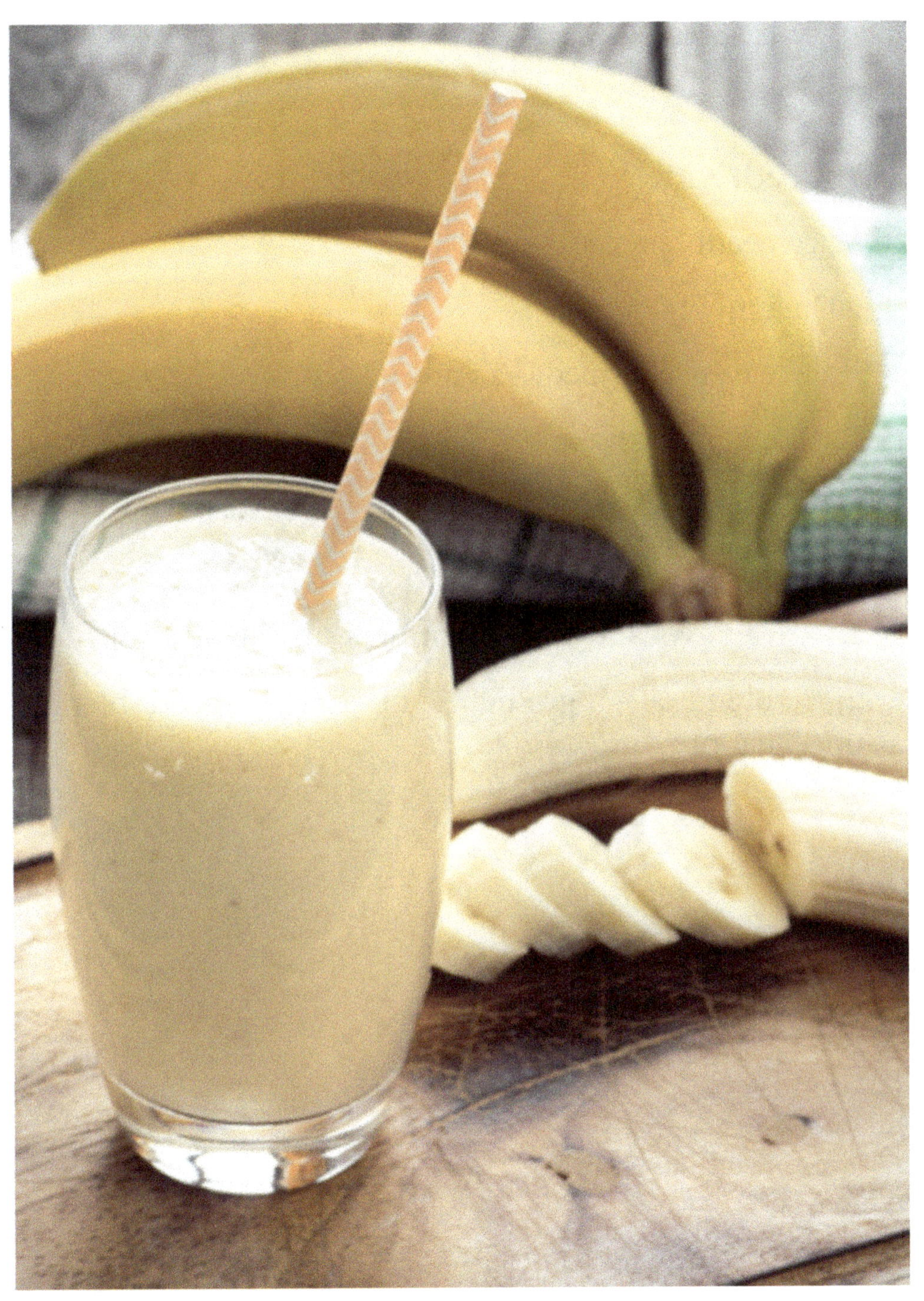

Detox Smoothie

Ingredients:

½ Avocado, peeled, pitted

2 Cucumbers

Kale leaves, chopped, ½ cup

Basil, about 4 leaves

Instructions:

1.	Cut avocado and cucumbers for the blender.

2.	Blend all ingredients in a high-speed blender until smooth.

3.	Enjoy!

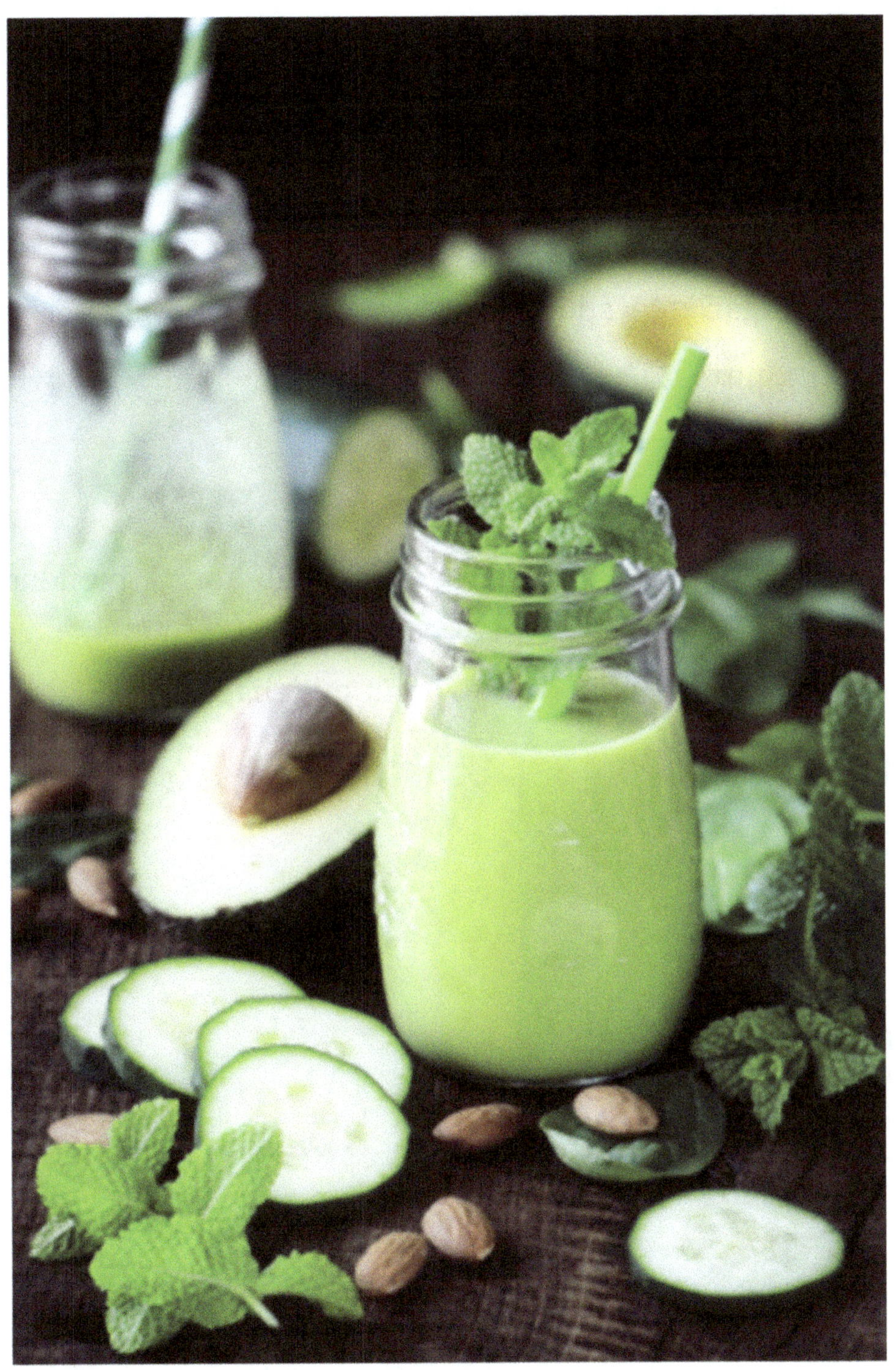

Plum and Grape Smoothie

Ingredients:

Grapes (Seeded), ½ cup

Date Sugar, 2 teaspoons

Plums, pitted, ½ cup

Instructions:

1.   Blend all ingredients in a high-speed blender until smooth.

2.   Pour the mixture into a nut milk bag.

3.   Enjoy!

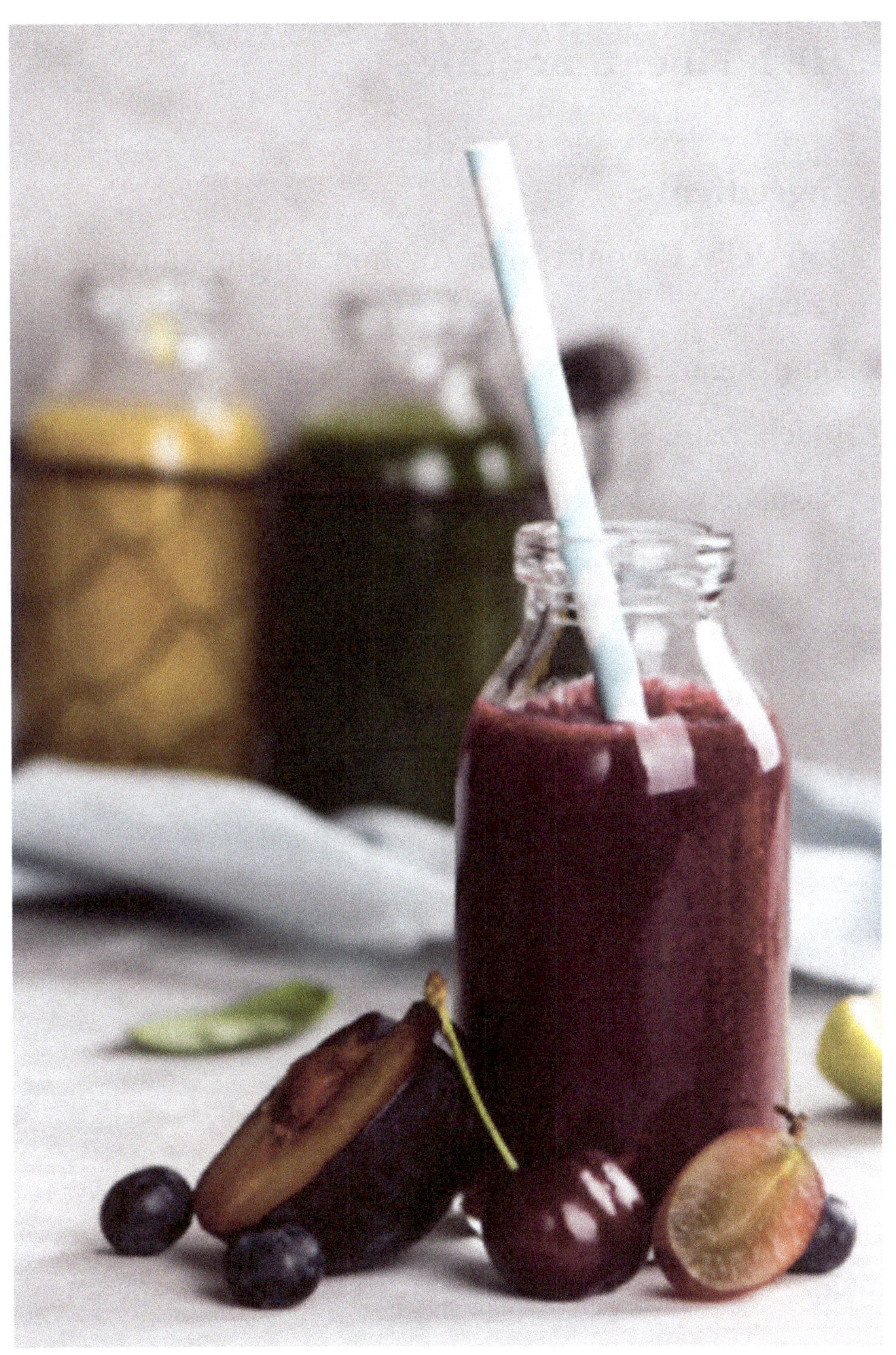

High Fiber Smoothie

Ingredients:

Soft Jelly Coconut Milk (or homemade walnut milk), ½ cup

Date Sugar, 2 teaspoons

Blueberries, ¼ cup

Raspberries, ¼ cup

Raw Sesame Seeds, 2 tablespoon

Instructions:

1.   Blend all ingredients in a high-speed blender until smooth.

2.   Enjoy!

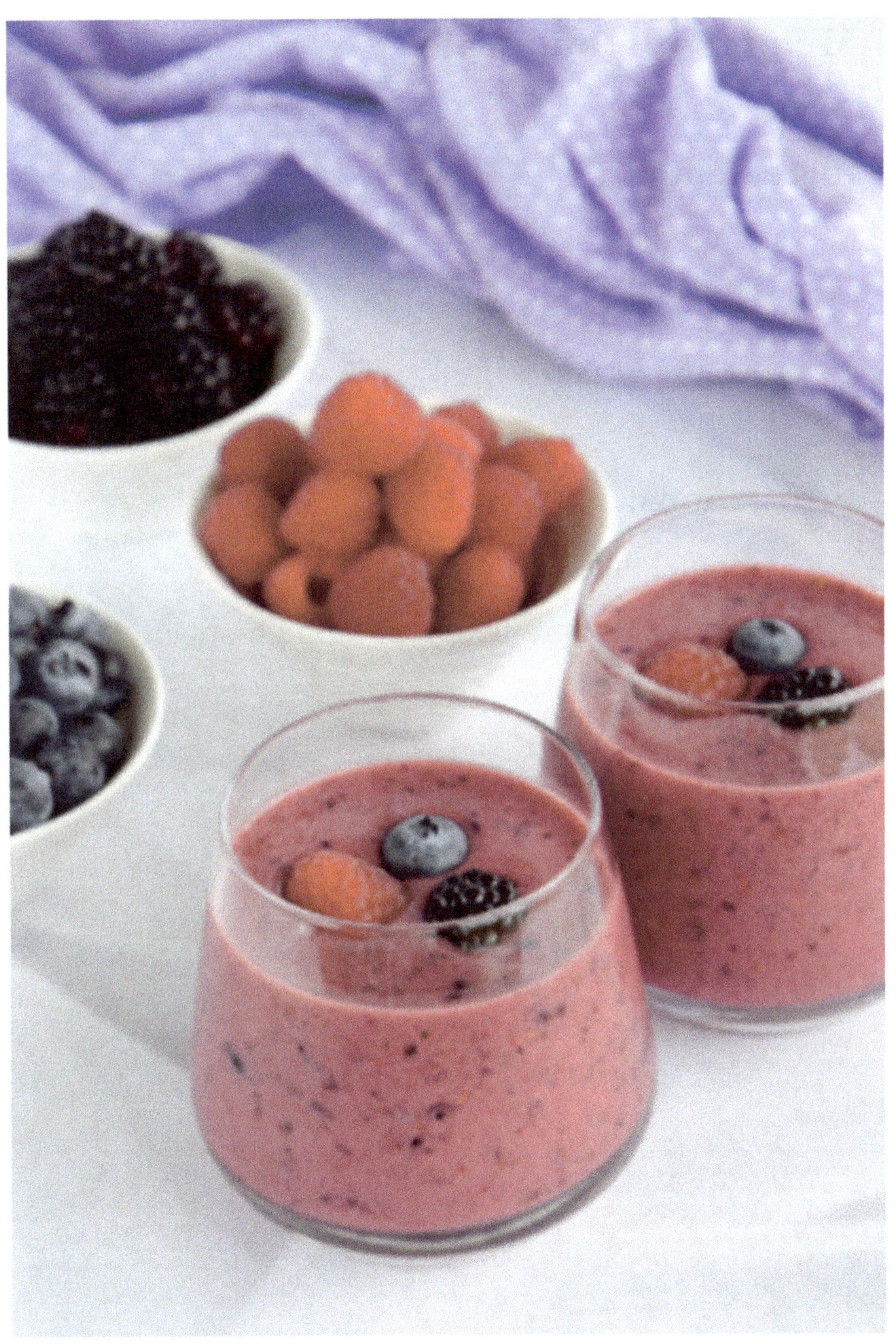

Melon Soul Smoothie

Ingredients:

Melons (Seeded), 6 oz (170

g)

Strawberries, ½ cup

Instructions:

1.   Cut melon for the blender.

2.   Blend all ingredients in a high-speed blender until smooth.

3.   Enjoy!

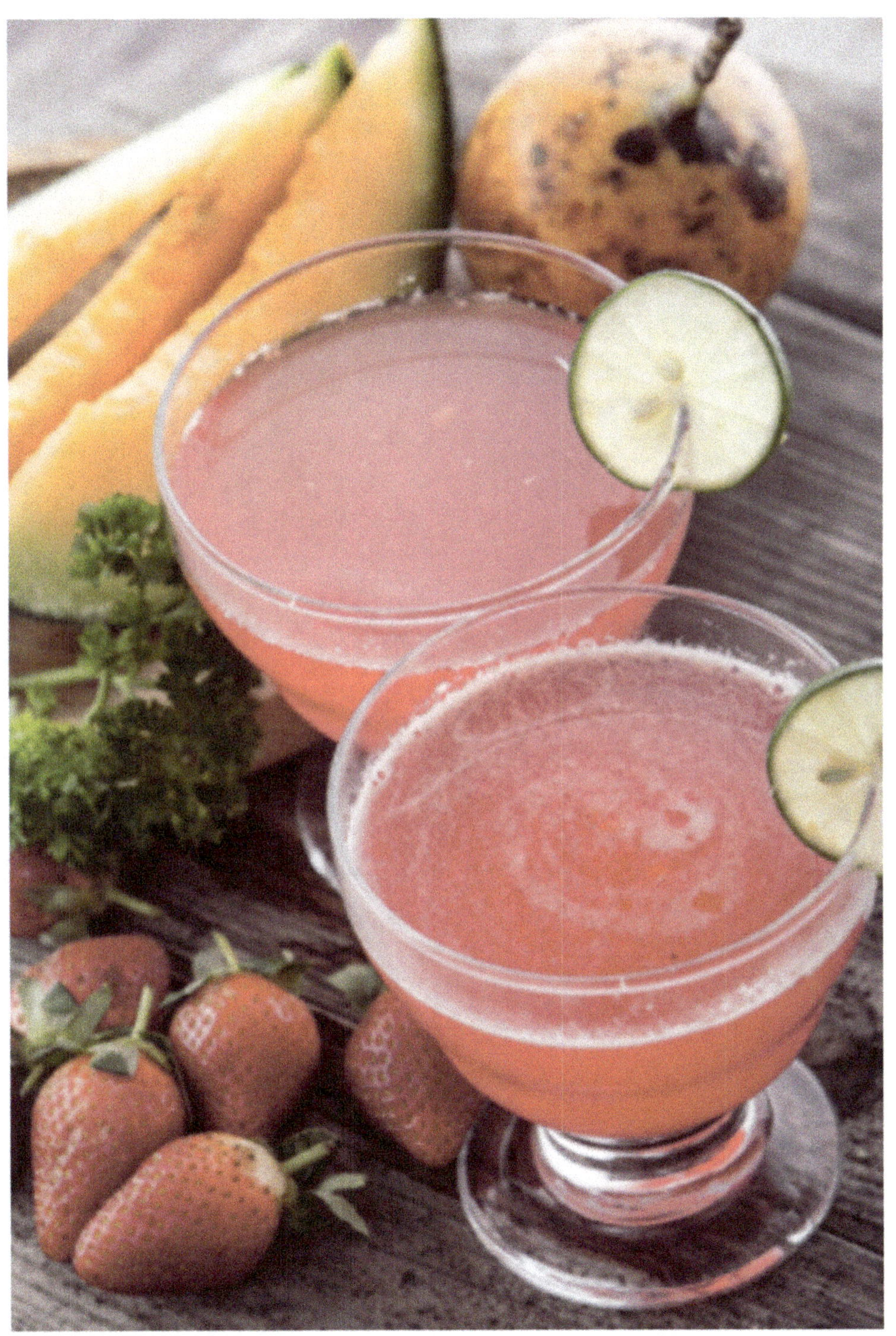